BTEC National Level 3

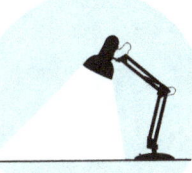

HEALTH & SOCIAL CARE (AAQ)

Revision Guide

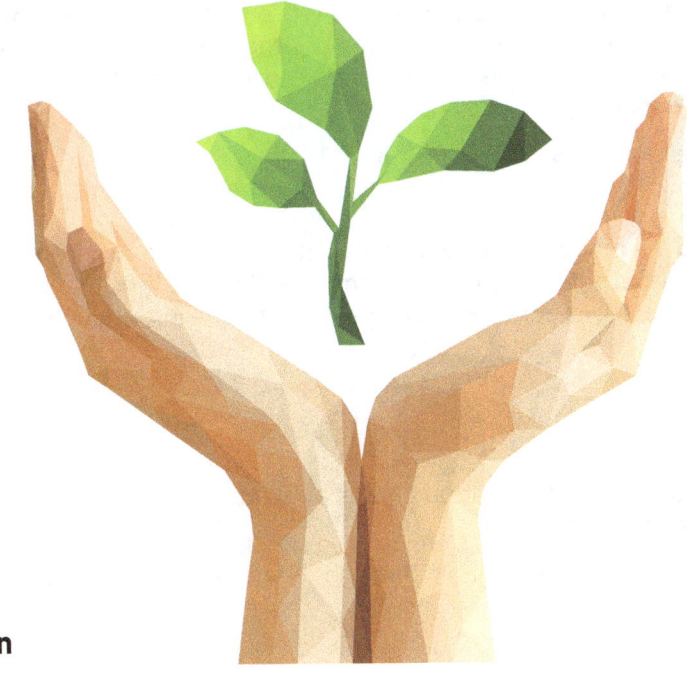

Hannah Long
Vicki Johnston

eboru

The publisher gratefully acknowledges the permission of copyright holders to reproduce copyright material.

Page 16: The Eatwell Guide is subject to Crown copyright protection, which is covered by an Open Government Licence. Source: OHID in association with the Welsh government, Food Standards Scotland and the Food Standards Agency in Northern Ireland.

Please see the remaining photo credits at: www.eboru.com/BTEC-HSC-RG-PhotoCredits

Cover image: © goodwin_x/Shutterstock

Every effort has been made to trace copyright holders and to obtain their permission for the use of copyright material. The publisher will be glad to make arrangements with any copyright holder it has not been possible to contact.

Copyright © 2025 Hannah Long, Vicki Johnston

All rights reserved. No part of this publication may be reproduced, distributed, or transmitted in any form or by any means, including photocopying, recording, or other electronic or mechanical methods, without the prior written permission of the publisher, or under licence from the Copyright Licensing Agency. See www.cla.co.uk for more details.

First edition 2025. Impression 10 9 8 7 6 5 4 3 2 1

ISBN 978-1-917048-05-7

Whilst every effort has been made to ensure all information in this book is correct, the publisher shall not be liable for any loss of profit or any other commercial damages, including but not limited to special, incidental, consequential, personal, or other damages, due to any information or advice contained in this book.

Ordering Information

Special discounts are available for class set purchases by schools, colleges and others. For details, contact the publisher at: orders@eboru.com

Trade orders: copies of this book are available through the normal wholesalers. For any queries please contact: orders@eboru.com

www.eboru.com

FEATURES IN THIS BOOK

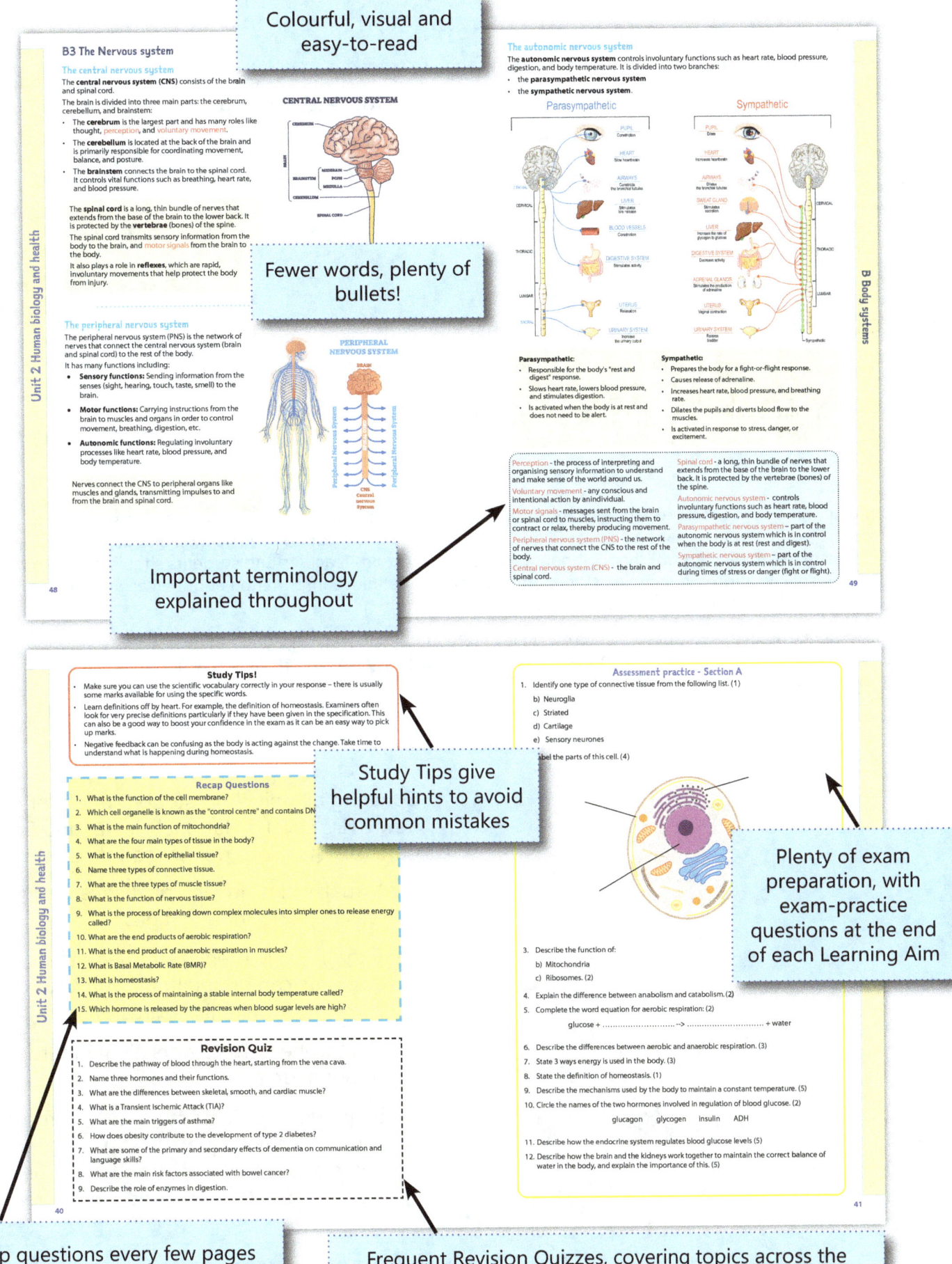

Contents

Unit 1 Human lifespan and development — 5
A Human growth and development through the life stages — 5
B Factors affecting human growth and development across each life stage — 14
C Health and social care promotion, prevention and treatment at different life stages — 25

Unit 2 Human biology and health — 39
A Organisation of the human body — 39
B Body systems — 46
C Disorders of the body and the effect on body systems — 69

Answers are available at: www.eboru.com/BTEC-HSC-RG-Answers

While this book is designed to help and support teachers and learners throughout the course the only official source of information about the qualification is the qualification specification and associated assessment guidance, published by the awarding organisation. Teachers and students should always refer to the specification and sample assessment material for definitive information about all aspects of this qualification. Specifications are also updated from time to time.

The practice questions, marks and answers included in this book are designed to help learners develop their knowledge, skills, understanding and technique but they do not replicate real examination papers, assessments or mark schemes.

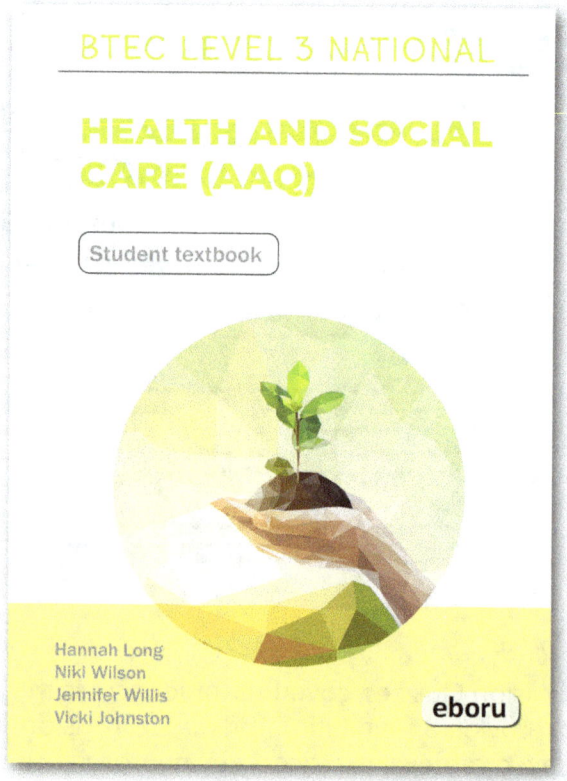

Covering all units, this student book for the new BTEC Level 3 National Health and Social Care (AAQ) is your perfect companion!

- **Visual:** Colourful and attractive design, with less text and more images
- **Engaging:** Written in language that students can understand, with keyword boxes for unfamiliar words on each spread
- **Comprehensive:** Covers all mandatory and optional units
- **Empowering:** Helps students to progress, with low-stakes questions for frequent recap and Case Studies and Activities to develop higher-level skills

ISBN: 978-1-917048-00-2

Unit 1 Human lifespan and development

A Human growth and development through the life stages

A1 Physical, Intellectual, Emotional and Social development at each life stage

Infancy

Infancy has an age range of **birth to 2 years**.

Physical

- **Rapid** growth and development occurs.
- **Growth** is indicated through physical measurements such as height, weight and head circumference.
- **Fine and gross motor skills** also develop.
  » Fine motor skill is the use of smaller muscles such as fingers and toes. E.g. pincer grip, holding a spoon and grasping small objects.
  » Gross motor skills are the use of larger muscles such as arms and legs. E.g. crawling, walking and lifting head up.

Intellectual

- A period of rapid intellectual growth.
- Infants learn by interacting with their environment. They become able to **recognise familiar faces** and **manipulate objects**.
- Language and communication rapidly develops from the age of 2 months.
  » 3 month olds can babble, make noises and recognise familiar voices.
  » 12 month olds can copy sounds and say simple words like 'dada'.
  » 2 year olds can say simple phrases and most will know 200-500 words, even if they can't say them all.

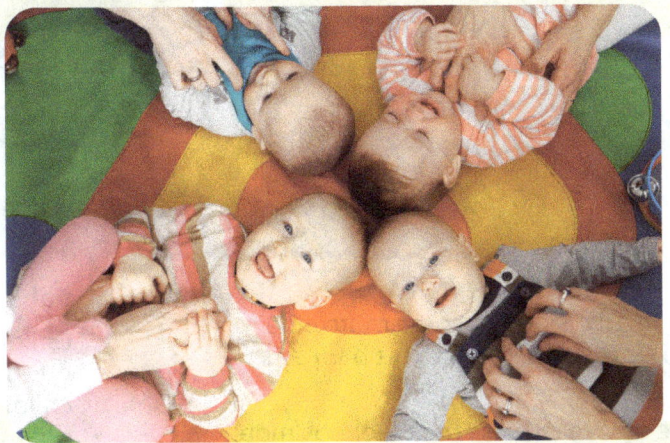

Emotional

Bonding and attachment refer to a strong emotional connection between an infant and their main caregiver(s).

- **Bowlby's** theory of attachment states that infants have an **innate ability** to form a positive attachment with a **primary caregiver** during the **critical period** of infancy.
- **Ainsworth's** theory of attachment identified **three attachment types** based on her **Strange Situation Study**. These attachment types are linked to the quality of caregiving.
  » **Secure** – when infants displayed signs of trust and feelings of safety with their caregiver. This is a sign of consistent and responsive caregiving.
  » **Anxious-resistant** – when infants displayed conflicting behaviours, as infants would seek proximity but then reject their mothers. This is a sign of inconsistent caregiving.
  » **Anxious-avoidant** – when infants did not display any form of closeness with the mother. This is a sign of unresponsive or emotionally distant caregiving.

Social

- Form relationships with caregivers through bonding and attachment.
- Begin to form relationships with other children through the **stages of play**.
  » **Solitary play** (0-18 months) where infants play on their own using their senses and the environment.
  » **Parallel play** (18-24 months) where infants will copy other children or adults and will play alongside others, but without sharing or turn-taking.

Early childhood

Early Childhood has an age range of **3-8 years.**

Physical

- **Growth** continues but at a slower rate compared to infancy and is heavily influenced by genetics and nutrition.
- Fine and gross motor skills continue to develop, and children can master certain skills at this point.

Examples include:
- Fine motor skills – doing up buttons and tying laces.
- Gross motor skills – riding a small bike and balancing on one foot by the age of 3.

Intellectual

Intellectual development typically occurs through sequential learning, where new skills build on existing ones.

- **Increase in vocabulary** – most children develop the ability to **talk in clear sentences** by the age of 4.
- Children **learn to count** and work with numbers.
- Their **problem-solving skills develop**.
- They know basic information about themselves such as their birthday and where they live.

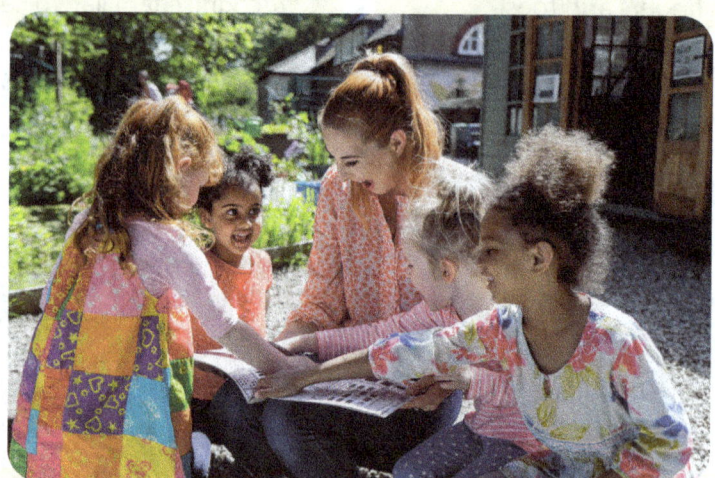

Emotional

- Children in this life stage become more able to **manage their own emotions**. This happens because:
  - They are able to express their feelings more clearly with language.
  - They are taught how to **regulate and name emotions** and given **coping strategies** for a range of emotions.
- They **develop their empathy skills**, so they can better understand others' feelings and emotions.
- **They develop their concept of 'self'.** This means they develop their identity and become able to identify aspects of their personality, such as 'I am nice'. These aspects become more complex towards the end of early childhood.

Social

- Children in this life stage are often surrounded by other children allowing them to **develop friendships.**
- Children often establish important friendships by the age of 7.
- Children widen their social circle through **co-operative play** as they learn to share and play alongside other children.

Adolescence

Adolescence has an age range of **9-18 years**.

Physical

Puberty is a period of rapid physical growth in adolescence. At the end of this life stage individuals will achieve sexual maturity.

- Puberty is stimulated by **sex hormones**. Primarily oestrogen and progesterone in females and testosterone in males.
- **Primary sexual characteristics** are those associated with the reproductive organs that were present from birth. For example, the uterus enlarges, the menstrual cycle begins, sperm production begins.
- **Secondary sexual characteristics** are outward physical that develop during puberty and signify adulthood. For example, pubic, armpit and facial hair and breast buds.

Intellectual

Adolescents develop an increased capacity for abstract thinking and reasoning. Both are crucial for problem solving.

- **Abstract thinking** involves concepts that are not directly linked to a real object or event. For example, time and justice are abstract concepts.
- **Reasoning skills** are when we can consider relevant facts and apply them logically, rationally and consistently.

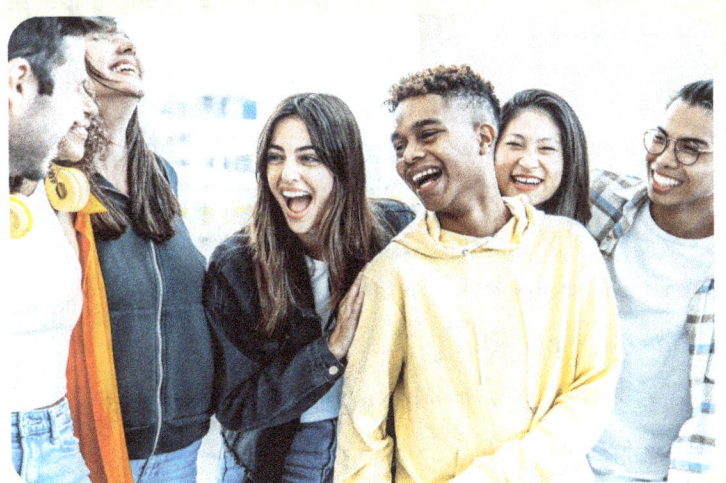

Emotional

- **Identity** continues to develop in this life stage as people have more external influences that contribute to the way they view themselves. For example, peer influences and social media.
- Identity helps to shape a person's **self-concept** including their self-image and self-esteem.
  » **Self-image** is a view of who we are, which includes our physical appearance and personality traits.
  » **Self-esteem** is an overall view of an individual's self-worth and confidence.
- **Intimate relationships** begin to develop in this life stage, as individuals start to explore their developing sexuality and closeness to others.

Social

By this life stage individuals will have an established social circle and will have **friendships** that they regularly choose to engage with.

- **Peer pressure** is when friends of a similar age influence decisions or behaviour. This can have positive or negative consequences.
- **Independence** develops throughout adolescence. People at 16 can choose to get a full-time job, people at 17 can learn to drive, and at 18 people legally become adults.

Study Tips!

- You need to know the names of each life stage and their age ranges.
- You need to know the PIES development of each life stage. Aim to know 2-3 examples of development for each area of PIES for each life stage.
- Where applicable you need to apply theories to the life stages. For example, Bowlby's attachment theory in infancy.

Important terms!

Growth – physical measurements of the body such as height and weight.

Development – the way in which things change, such as skills.

Fine motor skills – the use of smaller muscles such as those that control the fingers and toes.

Gross motor skills – the use of larger muscles such as those that control the arms and legs.

Attachment – the emotional bond between an infant and their primary caregiver.

Vocabulary – the range and number of words we know and use.

Primary sexual characteristics – present from birth and associated with our reproductive organs.

Secondary sexual characteristics – visible signs of physical change such as the development of breast buds or facial hair.

Abstract thinking – ability to think about concepts which can't be seen or touched.

Identity – how we view ourselves and our personality.

Self-concept – how we feel about the person we think we are. It encompasses our self-image and self-esteem.

Self-image – how we feel about the way we look.

Self-esteem – how we value ourselves.

Recap Questions

1. Give an example of a fine motor skill in infancy.
2. Who believes in the 'critical period'?
3. By what age does a child typically develop important friendships?
4. What are the stages of play in early childhood?
5. Name the main sex hormones responsible for puberty in a) males b) females.
6. Define the term 'self-esteem'.
7. Identify an example of social development in adolescence.
8. Who studied the Strange Situation?
9. Identify an example of intellectual development in infancy.
10. Give an example of a primary and secondary sexual characteristic.

Revision Quiz

1. What are two physical developments that are common in late adulthood?
2. What are two risk factors for breast cancer?
3. Name two lifestyle factors that can impact a pregnancy.
4. Why might a person's job affect their health?
5. Give two health conditions that are common in early childhood.
6. Describe the roles of two health care professionals that commonly work in hospitals.

Early adulthood

Early adulthood has an age range of **19-45 years**.

Physical

Individuals achieve **physical maturity** in this stage as puberty comes to an end and they stop growing.

- They reach **peak development** where an individual's height, strength and physical abilities are at their best and will not develop any further
- **Physical strength** peaks because muscles are at their strongest as the hormones that repair and grow muscle fibres are at optimal levels.
- Both men and women are at their most **fertile** in their 20s. Sex hormones are at their peak, meaning the quality of egg and sperm production is at its highest.
- Most **pregnancies** occur in this life stage. Hormonal changes in a woman's body support the pregnancy throughout, leading to a range of physical changes, including the suspension of menstrual cycles.
- **Lactation** is the production of milk for breastfeeding. The hormone prolactin stimulates milk production and oxytocin allows it to be released from the breast.
- The **brain continues to mature** until the mid-20s:
  » **Synaptic pruning** the removal of neural connections in the brain that are no longer needed, to improve efficiency.
  » The **prefrontal cortex** controls impulses and planning and is one of the last areas of the brain to develop.

Intellectual

- Earlier in this life stage people may continue to educate themselves in **higher** or **further education**. This further develops their intellectual abilities.
- People typically begin a long-term **career** in this life stage. This further develops their knowledge, skills and understanding.
- **Abstract thinking** becomes ever more refined as people apply their intellectual and life experiences to problems.

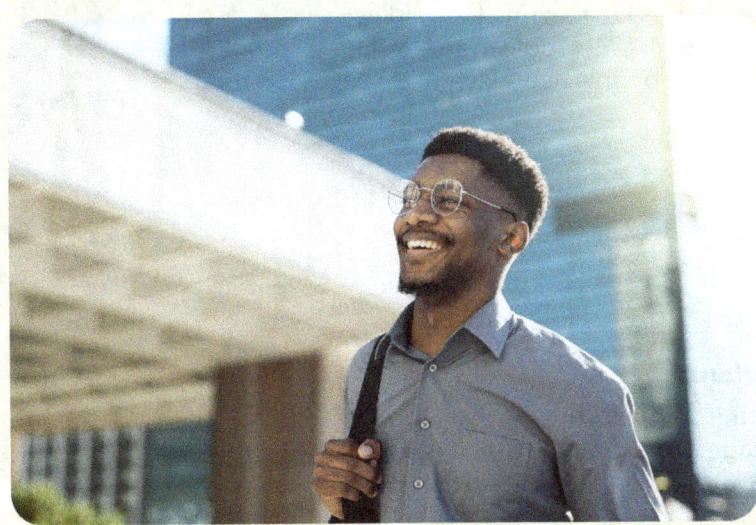

Emotional

- Adults in this life stage may enter into **long-term intimate relationships**.
- **Intimacy** refers to a deep and meaningful relationship with another person that can be displayed physically or emotionally.
- Life events, friendships, family and work commitments can **alter self-concept and self-image**, and affect **self-esteem**, in positive and negative ways. For example, people can start to view themselves differently due to establishing a career or becoming a parent.
- People begin to have their own children in this life stage, establishing new **bonds and attachments**.
- People's relationships with their own parents/guardians, siblings and other family can also develop.

Social

- Adults are at their most **independent** in this life stage.
  » They typically become fully financially independent from their family.
  » They often move out of the family home.
- Adults typically have an established **group of friends** but can develop more friends, for example, through work.

A Human growth and development through the life stages

Middle adulthood

Middle adulthood has an age range of **46-69 years**.

Physical

Women's fertile period comes to an end.

- » **Perimenopause** is the stage before menopause, when fertility declines. It is indicated by a change in menstruation and ovulation, as the ovaries produce fewer eggs.
- » **Menopause** is reached when a woman has not had a period for 12 months. Common symptoms include hot flushes, night sweats and vaginal dryness.

Physical abilities start to decline:

- **Physical strength decreases** due to a loss of muscle mass.
- Eyesight and hearing decline. Many people need glasses in this life stage.

Lifestyle choices in the past can also begin to affect people:

- People begin to experience joint pain due to wear and tear.
- People tend to become less active and gain weight. Metabolism also reduces, meaning people need fewer calories.

Intellectual

- People have lots of life experience at this stage. This can lead to further **improvements in their verbal and reasoning skills.**
- This is because they have been able to **apply learning** and knowledge from a wide range of situations.

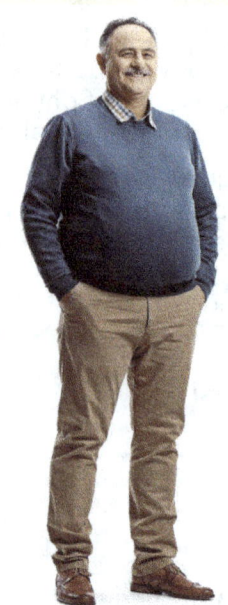

Emotional

- Adults towards the end of this life stage may begin to **re-evaluate their priorities** as changes in their circumstances may cause a shift in what they value most. For example:
  - » A change in work/life balance.
  - » A desire to achieve some particular goals.
- They may experience **empty nest syndrome** – when an adult experiences feelings of emptiness and loneliness because their children have left the family home.
- Individuals may also experience **emotional reactions** to changes in physical health such as:
  - » Low mood and loss of libido due to menopause.
  - » A feeling of getting old.

Social

- Relationships and friendships with **peers at work** can deepen.
- As children grow up people in middle adulthood find they have fewer responsibilities and more time than for many years.
- Retirement towards the end of this life stage, or early retirement can increase social opportunities and lead to a more active **social life**.
- However, some individuals may have a more **limited social life** due to changes in physical health, work pressures.
- People's social roles also change – at this age some become grandparents.

Late adulthood

Late Adulthood has an age range of **70-84 years.**

Physical
- **Reduction of lung capacity.** A loss of elasticity in the lungs impacts the body's ability to exchange take up oxygen and remove carbon dioxide.
- **Arteries and heart muscles thicken** which is known as arteriosclerosis. This can lead to hypertension (high blood pressure) and increases the risk of stroke and heart attack.
- **Brain cells lose some function** as neurons and other brain cells can die, shrink or lose connections to each other.
    » This can lead to a decline in brain function.
    » However it is a gradual process and the brain can adapt to the changes, meaning there is no noticeable change in many people.
- A decline in muscle mass and strength leads to **reduced mobility** and increased risk of falls and further complications such as broken bones.

Intellectual
- The physical decline of the brain makes it harder to learn new skills and information.
- Short-term memory declines, making it harder to recall recent information.
- However, older adults' wisdom and creativity remains intact.

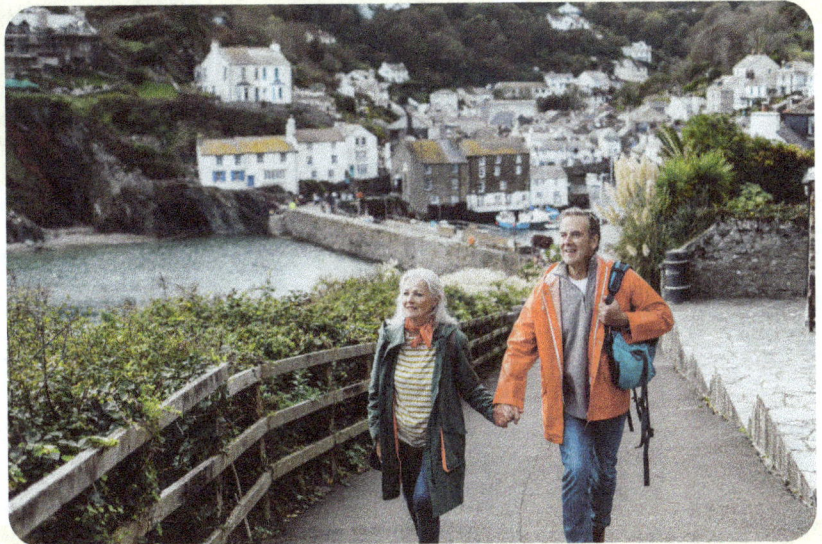

Emotional
- Late adulthood can be a time of **calmness** as adults become more at peace with themselves and their life.
- As with some other life stages, people in good health may feel younger than they actually are.
- Negative emotions may also appear such as feelings of **loneliness**, feeling **frail** and issues with existential security.

Social
- Retirement is very likely for anyone in this life stage that has not already retired. This can mean an individual has:
    » **more social opportunities** for meeting friends
    » more time for new hobbies and meeting new people.
- However, the loss of friends and family (bereavement) can **reduce the social circle**.

A Human growth and development through the life stages

Later adulthood

Later adulthood has an age range of **85+ years.**

Physical

Health continues to decline in this life stage.

- **Reduction in organ function** as cells and tissues in the body become less efficient. For example, the kidneys lose the ability to filter efficiently and have greater difficulty removing waste.
- **Bone density declines** leading to osteoporosis and brittle bones.
- Joints can become stiff as **ligaments and tendons lose elasticity**, causing stiffness and reduced mobility.
- Skin becomes **thinner and loses elasticity**, due to a lack of collagen, elastin and fat.
- **Chronic and long-term health conditions** become more likely. For example issues with immunity, cardiovascular disease and COPD.
- **Vision and hearing** can deteriorate quite badly.

Intellectual

- **Memory function** continue to decline from middle and late adulthood, due to the physical changes in the brain.
- Further **cognitive decline** can occur due to health issues such as a **stroke** or **dementia**. These conditions cause parts of the brain to become ineffective.
- **Cognitive super-agers** are when an individual's cognitive abilities remain intact and show no signs of decline. This occurs for a variety of reasons such as positive lifestyle choices, good emotional regulation and good brain structure.

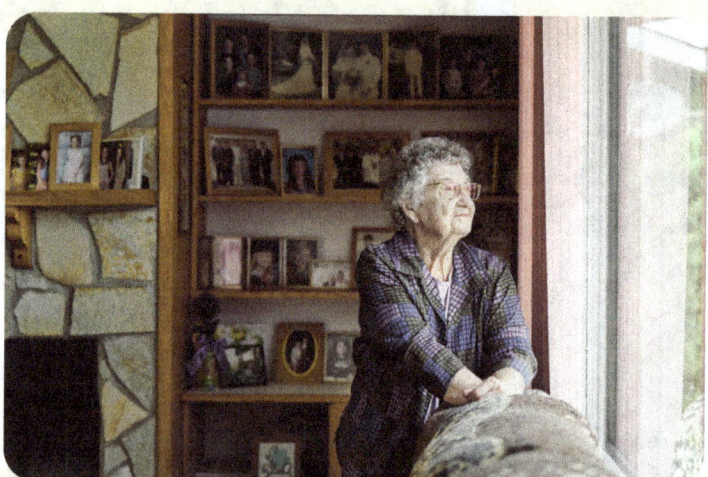

Emotional

- Individuals can have **improved emotional regulation** as they become reflective on their life and experiences and focus on positive experiences.
- However people can suffer **depression** linked to bereavement and loss of independence and skills.
- People have a strong **awareness of their own mortality and frailty** which can be associated with negative emotions.

Social

- There is a **reduction in social activity** due to further physical decline and loss of friends and social circles.
- **Increased need for support** from others to be able to meet friends and family outside of the home.
- **Social disengagement theory**, proposed by Cummings and Henry in 1961, argues that individuals naturally disengage from society as a part of the ageing process and become more relaxed without the need for a social life.
- **Activity theory**, proposed by Havighurst in 1961, contradicts disengagement theory as he argues that individuals have a shift in their social role and can become more social due to adapting to their current lifestyle. For example, retirement may see a change in responsibilities within the family or work.

Study Tips!
- You need to understand the key differences between the life stages particularly late adulthood and later adulthood.
- You need to be able to give relevant examples of health issues when explaining key points.

Important terms!

Physical maturity – when the body has fully developed or matured.

Peak development – when the body's physical functions have reached their maximum performance level.

Synaptic pruning – when the brain remove neurons and other cells in the brain that are no longer needed, to improve efficiency.

Intimacy – an emotional connection between two or more individuals that can be physical and emotional.

Retirement – a life event where an individual no longer works.

Bereavement – a life event where an individual loses a loved one.

Collagen – a protein in the body that provides structure to the skin.

Elastin – a protein in the body that provides elasticity to organs.

Hypertension – high blood pressure due to narrowed arteries.

Arteriosclerosis – the condition where arteries become harder and ticker. (Note that 'atherosclerosis' is a type of arteriosclerosis due to a build up of plaque.)

Existential security – a feeling of safety in a person's mortality.

Recap Questions

1. State the age range of late adulthood.
2. Which theory believes an individual naturally withdraws from society?
3. Identify an example of emotional development in early adulthood.
4. In later adulthood, skin loses elasticity due to a lack of which proteins?
5. Define the term 'cognitive super-agers'.
6. Which life stage may experience perimenopause?

Assessment practice

1. Give one example of a secondary sexual characteristic in a female. (1)
2. State three physical changes during puberty for a female. (3)
3. State a definition of abstract thinking. (1)
4. Identify an example of a gross motor skill in infancy. (1)
5. Identify a theory of attachment. (1)
6. State a definition of self-esteem. (1)
7. Identify two physical changes in later adulthood. (2)
8. Steve is 32 years old. State two previous life stages Steve has gone through including the age ranges. (2)
9. Give an example of intellectual development in early adulthood. (1)
10. Explain how peer pressure in adolescence could influence physical development. (4)
11. Outline one way to improve intellectual development in early childhood. (2)
12. Discuss the importance of attachment in infancy and early childhood. (9)

B Factors affecting human growth and development across each life stage

B Factors affecting human growth and development across each life stage

B1 Genetic factors
- Genes are made up of DNA (Deoxyribonucleic acid).
- DNA controls development of the body.
- Our genes/DNA are **inherited** from biological parents through 23 pairs of chromosomes.
- Genetics influences physical traits such as height, eye colour and hair colour.

Genetic predisposition
- A **genetic predisposition** refers to an increased likelihood of developing a health condition because of our genes.
- However, it does not mean that someone will definitely develop the health condition.
- In addition, many conditions can also be caused by environmental and lifestyle factors.
- Examples of genetically predisposed conditions include cardiovascular disease, cancer, obesity and mental ill health.

Cardiovascular disease
- A broad term for a range of conditions that affect the heart and blood vessels.
- A genetic variation known as **chr9p21** means an individual is at increased risk of inflamed blood vessels.
- Inflammation contributes to a build-up of deposits in the arteries which leads to **hypertension**.
- Hypertension can result in a stroke or heart attack.

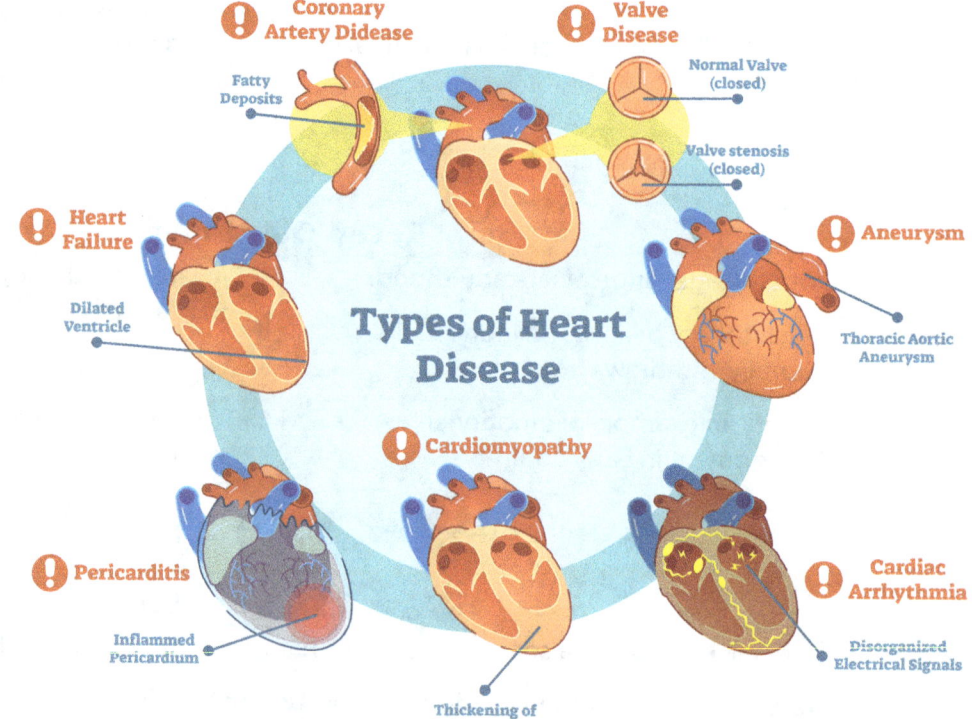

Breast and prostate cancer
- Breast cancer is most common in females but can also affect males.
  » Cells in the breast grow abnormally to form tumours.
- Prostate becomes enlarged and affects the function of the urethra.
  » Symptoms include difficulty or frequent urination.
  » The risk of prostate cancer increases if a close family member has the condition.

The gene known as **BRCA1** or **BRCA2** raises the risk of breast or prostate cancer.

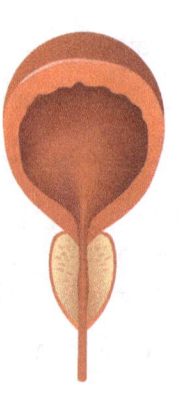
Healthy prostate

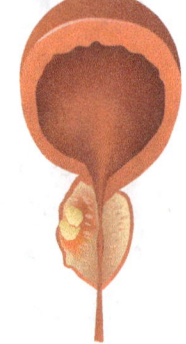
Prostate cancer

Genetic disorders

Genetic disorders are conditions inherited from one or both biological parents due to a faulty gene.

Huntington's disease

- A neurodegenerative disorder that stops parts of the brain from functioning over time.
- Everyone has two copies of the **HTT gene**, each inherited from a different parent. If one of them is faulty then you will develop the condition.
  » If one parent has the faulty gene then there is a 50% chance a child will have the condition.
  » If both parents have the faulty gene then there is a 75% chance a child will have the condition.
- Because someone only needs one copy of a faulty HTT gene to develop, it is called a **dominant gene**.
- Symptoms include mood swings, personality changes, memory loss, reduced mobility and difficulty swallowing and speaking.
- There are treatments but there is no cure.

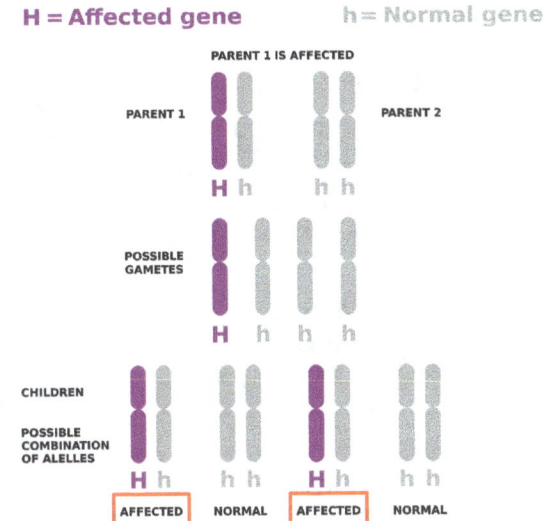

Cystic fibrosis

- CF is a disorder that causes breathing difficulties.
- It is caused if a child inherits two copies of the mutated CFTR gene, one from each biological parent.
  » If both parents carry the faulty gene, but do not have the condition, then there is 25% chance of a child developing it.
  » Because someone needs two copies of the faulty gene to develop CF, it is called a **recessive gene** (and a recessive disorder.)
- Symptoms include a thick sticky mucus in the lungs causing shortness of breath and a cough.
- Managed through medications, physiotherapy and exercise.
- Typically diagnosed in newborns using the heel prick test.
- There is no current cure.

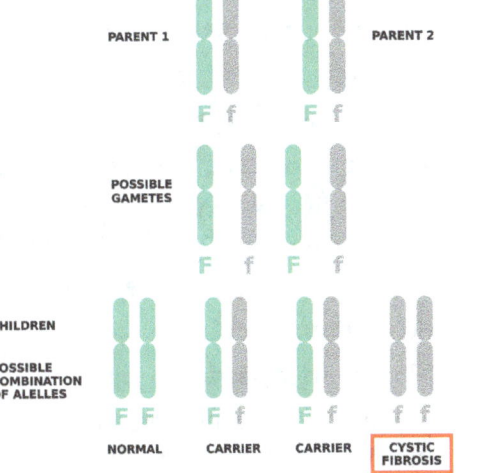

Sickle Cell Anaemia

- A faulty gene must be inherited from both biological parents for sickle cell to develop.
  » If both parents carry the faulty gene, but do not have the condition, then there is 25% chance of a child developing it.
  » Just as with CF, sickle cell is a recessive disorder.
- The condition affects haemoglobin, causing red blood cells to change shape and become clumped together. This causes blockages in blood vessels which can cause severe pain.
- It requires ongoing treatment from a multi-disciplinary team to prevent and reduce sickle cell crises.

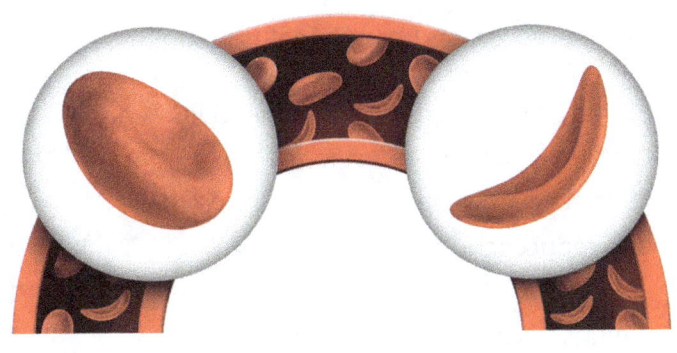

B2 Lifestyle factors

A lifestyle factor is something an individual **chooses** to do. For example, smoke or take regular exercise.

Diet and weight management

- A healthy diet should follow the NHS's Eatwell Guide. It recommends:
  » Adult men consume 2500 kcal
  » Adult women consume 2000 kcal per day.
- A calorie surplus is when you consume more calories than your body needs.
- A calorie deficit is when you consume fewer calories than your body needs.

The Eatwell Guide ensures that your body gets the right amount of all the nutrients it needs to be healthy.

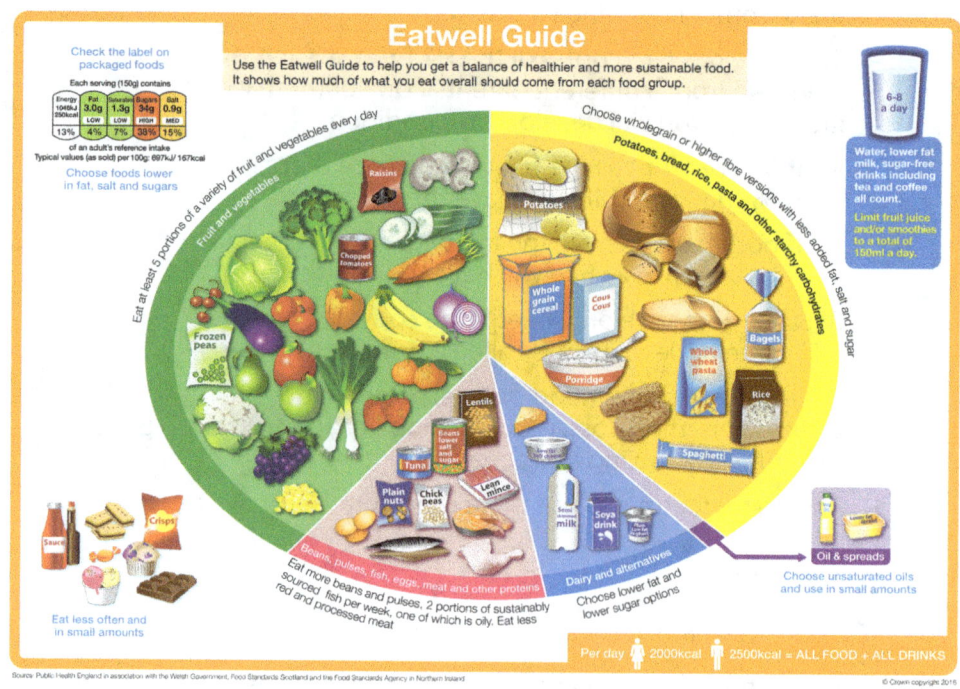

A healthy diet supports the maintenance of a healthy weight which contributes to:

- » A strong immune system
- » Positive self-image
- » Greater mobility and stronger joints
- » Greater ease of exercise
- » The prevention of long term health conditions

- An unhealthy diet can mean a calorie surplus or deficit, or the wrong proportion of nutrients, such as too many unhealthy fats or not enough fibre.
- An unhealthy can lead to health problems such as:
  » Malnutrition or obesity
  » Poor mobility/strained joints
  » Increased risk of numerous health conditions including: cardiovascular disease, diabetes, strokes, dementia and various cancers.

Level of exercise

Regular exercise has lots of benefits for holistic health and wellbeing:

- Strengthens heart, bones and muscles.
- Improves self-image/esteem.
- Social opportunities

It also reduces the risks of:

- Obesity.
- Injury, because muscles are stronger.
- Type 2 diabetes.
- Hypertension.
- Cardiovascular disease.
- Certain types of cancers.
- Joint and back pain.

The UK's Chief Medical Officer recommends: the average healthy adult should:

- Do at least 150 minutes of moderate or 75 minutes of vigorous physical activity, every week.
- Be active every day.
- Do muscle-strengthening exercises at least twice per week.
- Minimise periods of inactivity and sitting down.

- Depression.
- Osteoporosis.

There are also other benefits:

- Better sleep.
- Reduced stress.
- Helps maintain a healthy weight.

Alcohol

The department of health recommend that adults consume no more than 14 units of alcohol per week.

- Higher levels of alcohol consumption are associated with issues such as cirrhosis, heart disease, hypertension, strokes, liver disease and various cancers.
- People should also avoid binge drinking even if they drink less than 14 units per week.
- Alcohol affects the development of a foetus, so pregnant women should not drink alcohol.

As well as long-term health risks, alcohol affects decision making and leads to riskier behaviour such as: accidents, drink-driving and unprotected sex.

It also strongly linked to increased levels of violence and domestic abuse.

Tobacco

Tobacco use causes cancer.

- Cigarette smoke contains carcinogens which causes cells to mutate, leading to cancerous tumours.
    » Smoking is associated with numerous cancers including lung, mouth and throat.
- Smoking is also linked to other health issues such as heart disease, COPD (emphysema and bronchitis), dementia and strokes.
- Pregnant women should not smoke as it can damage the development of the foetus.
- Passive smoking can also be a risk to others, particularly those with respiratory conditions or pregnant women.

Quality of sleep

The recommended amount of sleep for an adult is between 7-9 hours per night. Sleep is needed to:

- Repair cells
- Restore energy
- Improve cognitive functioning.

Sleep deprivation and insomnia can lead to physical and mental health issues such as:

- » A weaker immune system, difficulty in concentrating, hypertension, heart disease, strokes, obesity and type 2 diabetes.
- Other lifestyle factors can influence the quality of sleep, such as exercise, diet and substance use.

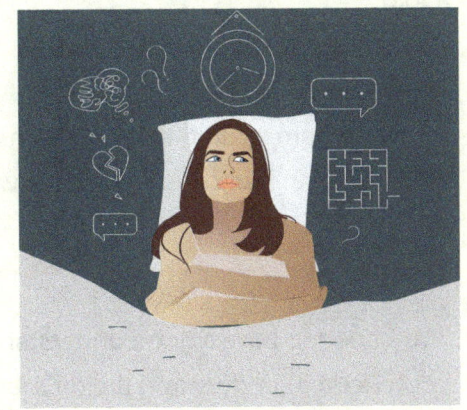

Oral health

Regular teeth and gum cleaning helps to keep a person's mouth and teeth clean and healthy.

Good oral health routines for adults means:

- Brushing teeth twice a day, flossing, and using mouthwash.
- A healthy mouth and teeth can improve a person's self-image and self-esteem as they feel good in their appearance.

Poor oral health leads to lead to bad breath, gum disease and tooth decay.

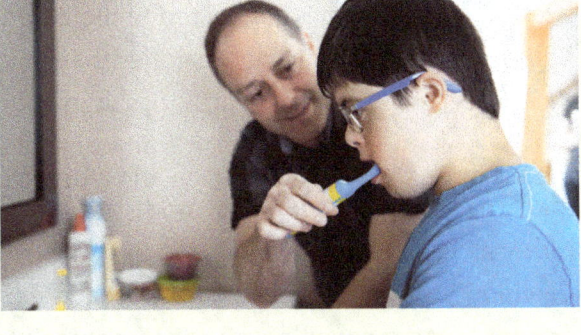

- If teeth are not cleaned regularly, bacteria in the mouth feed on remains of food to produce acid which attacks teeth, eventually creating holes and decay.
- A sugary diet and alcohol consumption can speed up this process.
- Smoking has a negative effect on overall oral health, including an increased risk of gum disease and mouth and throat cancer.

B Factors affecting human growth and development across each life stage

Pregnancy

Lifestyle factors contribute to a healthy pregnancy and the development of the foetus. Pregnant women should:

- Avoid alcohol, tobacco and recreational drugs. All of these can:
  - » pose serious health risks to an unborn baby
  - » cause premature birth.

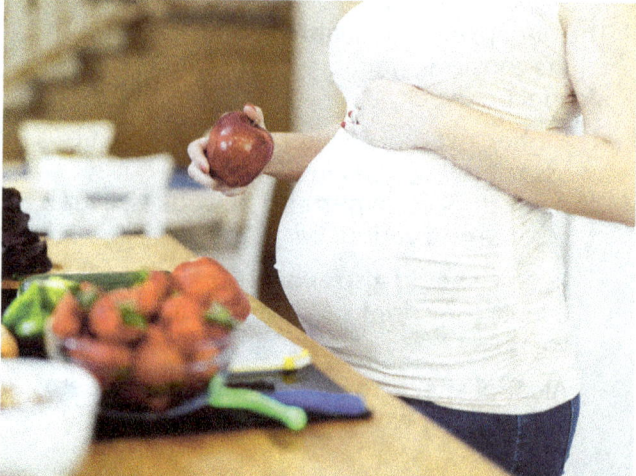

- Follow a healthy diet, to ensure both mother and baby are receiving the correct nutrients in the right quantities. This supports the growth and development of the foetus.
- A healthy diet is generally the same as for any adult but with the following differences:
  - » **Folic acid** supplements are recommended before conception and for the first 12 weeks of pregnancy. This supports the early-stage development of the foetus.
  - » More protein is needed, to power growth and repair.
  - » Ensure there are no deficiencies in vitamin D, calcium or iron.
  - » Two portions of oily fish per week – but no more than two.
- Avoid:
  - » raw fish, shark, swordfish, marlin
  - » raw eggs
  - » pâtés, game, cured meat and fish
  - » more than four cans of tuna per week.

> **Study Tips!**
> - You need to have a good understanding of the different types of genetic and lifestyle factors.
> - You need to understand the different types of genetic factors and the impact these can have upon development.

> **Important terms!**
> Urethra – a tube that is connected to the bladder which allows urine to pass through.
> Calorie surplus – eating more calories than your body needs each day.
> Calorie deficit – eating fewer calories than your body needs each day.
> Binge drinking – consuming large amounts of alcohol in a short amount of time. 'Large amounts' means more than 8 units for men and 6 units for women in a single session. This is roughly 4 pints for men, 3 pints for women, of moderate strength (4%) beer.
> Cirrhosis – scarring of liver tissue which causes permanent damage to the function of the liver.
> Carcinogens – cancer-causing toxins that are present in tobacco smoke.
> Emphysema – a condition caused by damage to the walls of the alveoli in the lungs that leads to shortness of breath and coughing.
> Passive smoking – breathing in second-hand smoke from a nearby smoker.
> Sleep deprivation – not getting the recommended amount of sleep per night.
> Insomnia – a condition that prevents a person getting to sleep or staying asleep.

Recap Questions

1. Identify a symptom of cystic fibrosis.
2. Identify a negative effect of not exercising.
3. Give an example of a lifestyle factor that can impact foetal development in pregnancy.
4. What is the condition that causes abnormally-shaped red blood cells?
5. How many hours of sleep is recommended per night?
6. Identify a physical health issue related to tobacco use.
7. Give an example of a lifestyle factor that could impact the amount of sleep a person has.
8. Give a negative effect of not regularly brushing teeth.
9. Identify a prenatal vitamin that supports foetal development in pregnancy.

Revision Quiz

1. Describe one attachment type described by Ainsworth in her Strange Situation Study.
2. Describe two common emotional developments in adolescence.
3. What impact can menopause have on physical and emotional development?
4. Explain the term 'genetic disposition'.
5. Give one example of a health inequality due to socioeconomic status.
6. Why do people with a learning disability experience inequalities in access to health services?
7. What are the main features of meningitis?
8. Which life stages are most prone to obesity?
9. Describe the concept of 'herd immunity'.
10. Describe the role of a speech therapist. What age range do they typically work with?
11. Outline the main features of an integrated care system.
12. Why is quality of sleep important for health and wellbeing?

B Factors affecting human growth and development across each life stage

B3 Health inequalities

Current NHS definition of health inequalities

Health inequalities are defined by the NHS as:

> 'Unfair and avoidable differences in health across the population, and between different groups within society'

This definition recognises that there are differences in health outcomes across many different demographic groups. Different groups can have different experiences of the healthcare system, which can contribute to differences in health status and health outcomes.

Health inequality examples

Difference in life expectancy across different socioeconomic groups

Socioeconomic groups categorise people according to their social and economic positions.

- This covers things such as:
  » salary and wealth
  » type of job
  » level of education
  » social background

Average life expectancy in the UK in 2022 was 78.6 years for men and 82.6 years for women. However, this differs depending on where you live and your socioeconomic group.

- People in **managerial and professional jobs** tend to earn more, have more job security, with generous pensions, have better working conditions and have more control over their working life.
  » Examples of these types of jobs include: lawyers, doctors, IT project managers.
- People in **routine and service occupations** tend to be paid less, with less job security, smaller pensions, more hazardous working conditions, and with less control over their working life.
  » Examples of these types of jobs include: bar staff, labourers, lorry drivers.

The Office for National Statistics has found that on average:

- Men in the highest managerial and professional jobs live for over 5 years longer than those in more routine jobs, and for over 9 years longer than those who are long-term unemployed or who have never worked.
- For women the equivalent figures are 4 years and almost 6 years.

In addition, those who live in more deprived areas live shorter lives than those in more affluent areas.

- A postcode lottery impacts the amount of healthcare resources and services available to different groups of individuals.
- For example, those in a deprived area may experience more significant health concerns due to the unfair distribution of services and resources.

Prevalence of mental health difficulties

- Those who live in deprived areas often suffer more from mental health issues.
- People with less secure and less well-paid jobs are more likely to have mental health issues, such as anxiety and depression.
- This occurs for a variety of reasons such as:
  » financial difficulties
  » unemployment
  » poor housing
  » more limited access to services
  » a feeling of lack of control.

There are disparities for mental health issues according to **gender**.
- Females are more likely to suffer from anxiety or depression. They are, however, more likely to seek support compared to males.
- The male suicide rate is three times higher than the female suicide rate.
  - » This may be because of a perceived stigma attached to mental health and masculinity, meaning they do not seek help.
- Trans and gender-diverse people can face discrimination and stigma, which can cause mental health issues.

Race and **ethnicity** are also linked to mental health inequalities:
- The charity Mind reports that one in three people from racialised communities in the UK had experienced discrimination from mental health services.
- A larger percentage of Black people in the UK have experienced a mental health condition than white people.
- A disproportionate number of Black people in the UK are sectioned under the Mental Health Act compared to white people. However, Black people in majority Black countries do **not** have higher rates of mental health issues than white people in the UK.
  - » So, the reasons for these disproportionate numbers in the UK are **structural and social inequalities**.

Mental health inequalities linked to race and ethnicity are linked to a number of factors including:
- Inequalities in access to services
- Unconscious bias
- Services that are not designed to be culturally diverse
- Structural racism
- Personal experience of racism, discrimination and broader inequalities.

Access to health services

Location of services can impact a person's ability to attend a service. For example, if a service is far away and there is limited public transport, individuals may find it hard to attend appointments.

People with **learning disabilities** face large health inequalities.
- Women with a learning disability in the UK die on average 23 years earlier than women without a learning disability.
- For men the same figure is 19 years. (Source: 2022 Learning Disabilities Mortality Review).
- This is due to:
  - » A lack of accessible transport.
  - » Lack of understanding from professionals about learning disabilities.
  - » Professionals not recognising when someone has a learning disability.
  - » Incorrect diagnosis.
  - » Inadequate follow-up care.

Access to general healthcare services can depend on a person's **gender**:
- Healthcare systems, treatments and medicine have traditionally focused on men. This means that:
  - » Healthcare systems and professionals may sometimes misdiagnose women's symptoms and suggest less appropriate treatments.
  - » Female-only conditions, such as endometriosis, are more likely to be misdiagnosed.
  - » Women's symptoms are more likely to be dismissed.

Transgender and non-binary people are less likely to find services that are equipped to understand or meet their needs.

Just as with mental health services, **race and ethnicity** impacts people's access to general health services, for much the same reasons.

Discrimination

Although illegal under the Equality Act 2010 discrimination can still occur.

- Discrimination is defined as treating an individual or group of people unfairly because of a characteristic they possess.
- The nine protected characteristics under the Equality Act 2010 are: age, disability, gender reassignment, marriage and civil partnership, pregnancy and maternity, race, sexual orientation, sex.

If a person feels they have been discriminated against this leads to:

- a lower level of trust in the service
- lower rates of access to the service.

This then causes an increase in ill health and a decrease in positive health outcomes.

  » The NHS Race & Health Observatory reports that over half of Black, Asian and ethnic minority patients have experienced discrimination by a healthcare professional.

Environmental inequalities

The **environment** refers to an individual's surroundings There can be risks or hazards associated with the environment.

Exposure to pollution often occurs in urban areas where high levels of traffic emissions pollute the air.

- **Air pollution** increases the risk of developing health conditions such as:
  » respiratory diseases (including asthma)
  » cardiovascular disease
  » cancer.
- Noise and light pollution can also occur in urban areas, which can impact on mental health and cause sleep deprivation.

Unsafe housing conditions such as overcrowding or damp conditions can also increase health risks, including:

- **Asthma**
  » Pollutants from the air, pet hair or mouldy conditions can increase the chances of developing asthma.
  » Asthma rates are more prevalent amongst deprived areas and those from disadvantaged backgrounds.
- **Tuberculosis** (TB)
  » TB affects the lungs and is an infectious disease that is commonly spread through coughs and sneezes.
  » TB is easily spread in poor housing conditions, due to overcrowding.
  » Although TB rates remain low in the UK, they are still higher in urban areas
  » TB is more prevalent in people living in deprived areas.

Economic inequalities

Income and wealth has a big impact on health inequalities, along with employment status. People with a low income:

- Are more likely to suffer ill health conditions such as obesity, type 2 diabetes and asthma.
- Suffer higher average death rates from cancer.
- Find it harder to access health services and resources.
- Are less able to afford fresh food in order to maintain a healthy balanced diet.
- Are more likely to be in insecure, more physically demanding and more hazardous jobs.
- Are more likely to live in poorer-quality houses, in more polluted areas.
- Can't afford some costs associated with health.

Occupational-related health inequalities

Occupational health refers to health risks or conditions that are caused by a person's job.

Chronic obstructive pulmonary disorder (COPD) refers to a range of respiratory diseases, including emphysema and bronchitis

It can occur due to consistent exposure to pollutants such as dust, smoke and harmful chemicals

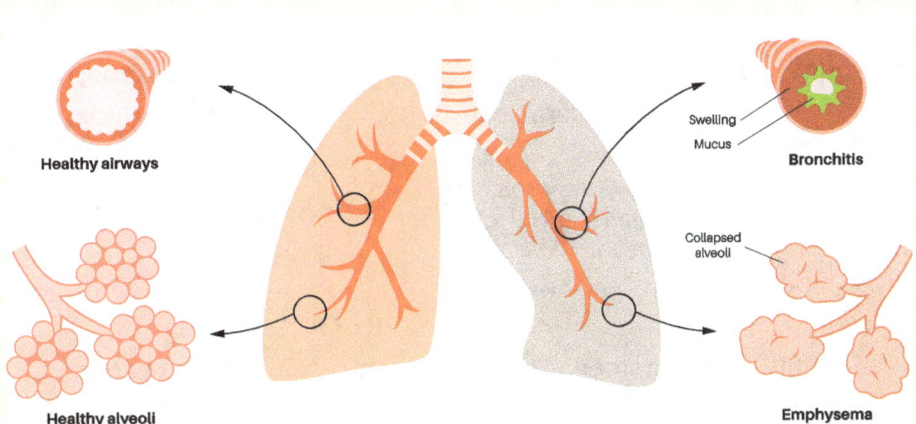

Musculoskeletal problems are issues that affect the joints or muscles.

- They typically occur if parts of the body are overworked for a long time – for example due to poor posture, lifting technique or lifting objects that are too heavy.
- They included back pain, joint pain and tendonitis
- Those with manual jobs are more likely to experience these issues.

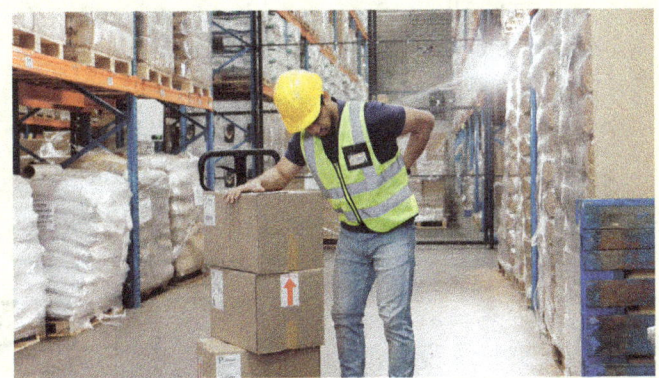

Stress and anxiety are common in the workplace.
 » Individuals may feel the pressure of workload, deadlines or conflicts with other people in the workplace.
 » The amount of stress and anxiety an individual suffers with will vary from person to person depending on their coping methods.

- **Shift work** is when a person works outside of the typical 9-5 working hours. This can include working evenings or night shifts.
 » Shift work interferes with our **circadian rhythm**, leading to sleep deprivation. This can lead to a range of health conditions.
 » Shift work can put a strain on personal relationships and limit social opportunities, leading to mental health problems.

For all these reasons, shift work leads to an increased risk of cardiovascular disease, type 2 diabetes, anxiety and depression, and possibly cancer.

Study Tips!
- You should be aware that the NHS definition of health inequalities could be updated at any time. So do check the most up to date definition on the NHS website.

Important terms!

Demographic groups – groups of individuals based on a similar characteristic or trait.

Health status – the overall condition of someone's health.

Health outcomes – the measurable results of healthcare.

Socioeconomic groups – a way to categorise people according to wealth and social status.

Postcode lottery – the differences in services and resources in different locations.

Discrimination – the unfair treatment of an individual or group of people based on a shared characteristic.

Tendonitis – a health condition in which tendons become inflamed due to consistent stress upon the joints.

Recap Questions

1. Identify an environmental factor that can lead to a health inequality.
2. Give an example of an occupational health condition.
3. Which gender is more likely to experience mental health difficulties without seeking support. Give a reason for your answer.
4. Define the term discrimination.
5. How does a postcode lottery lead to health inequalities?
6. How do economic factors influence health inequalities?
7. Identify a reason for a difference in life expectancy amongst different socioeconomic groups.
8. Identify a health condition because of environmental factors.

Revision Quiz

1. What emotional developments are common in early adulthood.
2. What is a 'cognitive super-ager'?
3. Describe the main features of cystic fibrosis.
4. At what life stage is stress at work most likely? Why?
5. What is the purpose of a vaccination?

Assessment practice

1. Explain how lifestyle factors can impact physical development. (4)
2. State what is meant by 'genetic predisposition'. (1)
3. Explain one way that environmental factors can contribute to health inequalities. (2)
4. a) Give an example of a genetic disorder. (1) b) Outline the main aspects of this disorder. (4)
5. Identify a health condition that is associated with occupational health inequalities. (1)
6. Outline the main impacts of poor oral health. (3)
7. State the current NHS definition of health inequalities. (1)
8. Explain how discrimination can lead to health inequalities. (2)
9. Discuss the impact that economic factors can have upon health inequalities. (9)

C Health and social care promotion, prevention and treatment at different life stages

C1 Prevalent health conditions

Infancy (0-2 years) and Early Childhood (3-8 years)

Flu (Influenza)

- A contagious viral condition that can cause symptoms such as:
  - fever
  - fatigue
  - dry cough
  - runny nose
  - ear pain.
- It is spread through coughs and sneezes.
- It can be serious and require hospital treatment.
- Mainly affects children under the age of five.

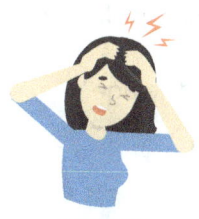
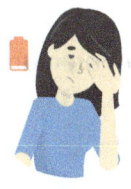
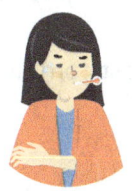
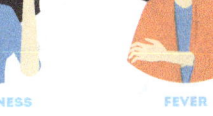
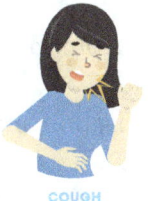
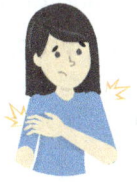
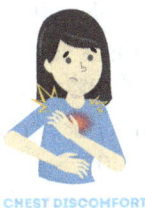

SYMPTOMS OF FLU: HEADACHE, WEAKNESS, FEVER, COUGH, MUSCLE ACHE, CHEST DISCOMFORT

Chicken pox

- A contagious condition that is transmitted via direct contact with an infected person, or via coughs and sneezes.
- Common symptom includes red spots or blisters across the body that can be itchy.
- Once a child has recovered from chicken pox they are immune from it for the rest of their life.
- Mainly affects children under the age of 10.

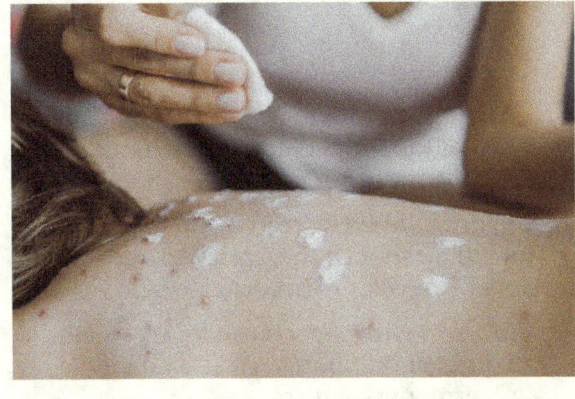

Ear infections

- Can be bacterial or viral.
- A common occurrence with other health conditions such as the flu.
- Symptoms include ear pain, sickness, high temperature, lethargy and hearing difficulties.
- Far more common in the middle ear, behind the ear drum.
- Children aged between six months and three years commonly develop ear infections.

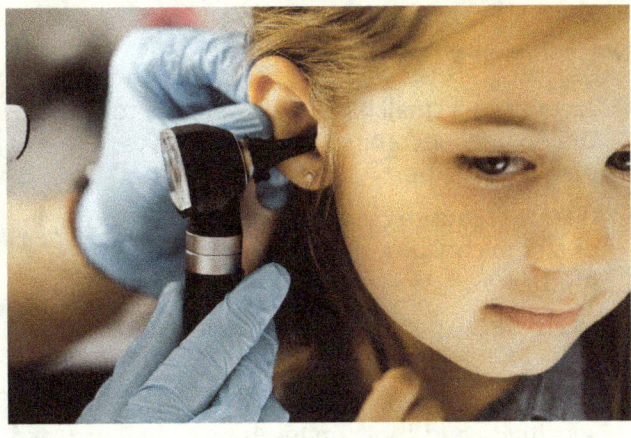

25

Meningitis

- Caused by inflammation of the protective membrane around the brain and spinal cord.
- Can be bacterial or viral.
- Symptoms include fever, headaches, nausea, vomiting, a rash that does not disappear when pressed, and possible seizures.
- Meningitis can be fatal and is a medical emergency.
- Most common in children under the age of 5.

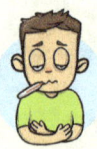 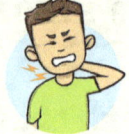 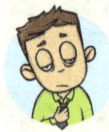
Fever — Neck pain — Sleepiness

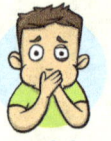 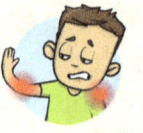 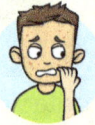
Vomiting — Joints pain — Rash

Conjunctivitis

- Highly contagious condition.
- Causes secretions or pus to release from the eye or eyes.
- This leads to redness, a burning sensation and itchiness.
- Can occur at any age.

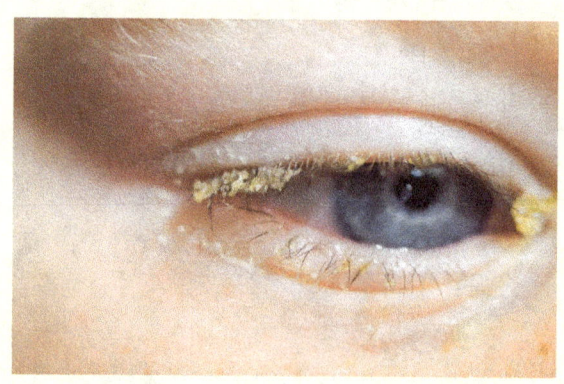

Speech development problems

- Normally identified around 12 months old if a child is not yet communicating verbally.
- Children are supported by professionals, including speech therapists, to address speech development problems.
- Problems with speech can be connected to other conditions, such as a hearing impairment or autism.

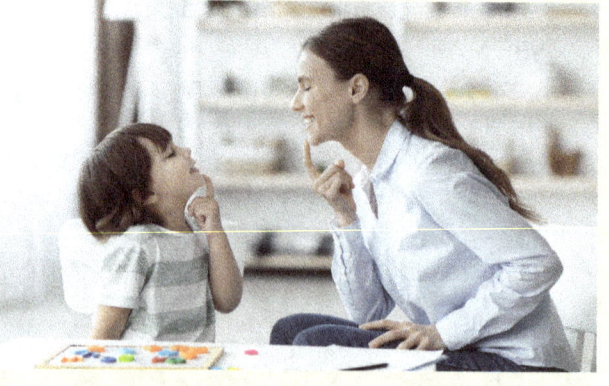

Dental caries (tooth decay)

- A **cavity** is a small hole in a tooth due to the enamel becoming damaged due to plaque build-up.
- Plaque is caused by poor oral hygiene and/or a high consumption of sugary drinks/food.
- Tooth decay gets worse if left untreated. This can result in teeth rotting.
- Symptoms include, tooth pain, teeth sensitivity and spots on teeth.
- Common in early childhood due to too many sweets, fizzy drinks etc.

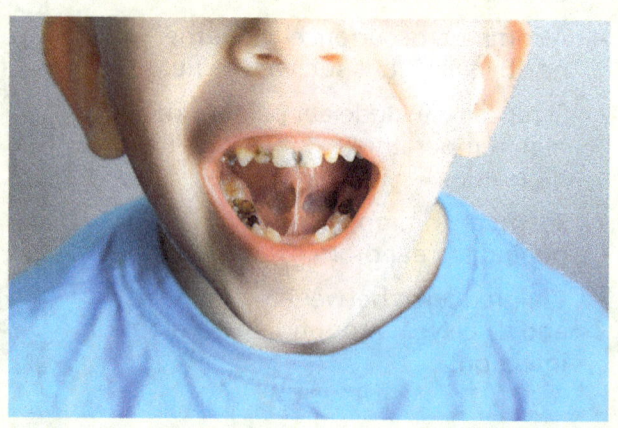

Adolescence (9-18 years)

Substance misuse

This includes **smoking, vaping, drugs and alcohol** use.

Adolescents can be influenced by peers to make risky lifestyle choices and behaviours.

- Smoking and vaping can lead to immediate health issues such as coughing and feeling out of breath.
    » Long-term effects include lung cancer, strokes, heart disease and emphysema.
- Alcohol can impact the development of the adolescent brain, leading to cognitive defects and delays.
    » Long-term health conditions include cirrhosis of the liver and increased risks of cancer and strokes.
    » Alcohol consumption can also lead to risky behaviour, leading to accidents, drink driving and sexual health issues, including sexually transmitted infections and unplanned pregnancies.
- Recreational drugs can damage organs, harm the development of the adolescent brain and cause mental health issues.
    » Addiction to illegal drugs can also cause social problems such as issues with school and family, and an increased risk of criminal activity.

Sexual health

- As adolescents' hormones change during puberty their interest in exploring sexual encounters increases.
- Without appropriate education about sexual health, adolescents are at risk of sexually transmitted infections or unplanned pregnancies.

Early adulthood (19-45 years) and middle adulthood (46-69 years)

Stress, depression and anxiety at work

- Balancing home life and a job can be demanding in these life stages and lead to additional pressures. For example, organising childcare around work patterns.
- Work pressure can lead to mental health issues such as stress, anxiety, depression and irritability. These can all lead to physical health issues.

Accidents from risk-taking behaviours

- Risky behaviour is more likely in very early adulthood and may include: reckless driving, risky lifestyle choices (e.g. drinking too much alcohol), extreme sports/activities and ignoring rules and regulations.
- This increases the risk of accidents which can lead to:
    » Acquired brain injuries
    » Life-altering injuries such as scars, burns, paralysis or loss of limbs.

Inactivity/sedentary lifestyle

- Individuals tend to gradually move around less as they get older.
    » This can be due to having a job where there is a lot of sitting down.
    » It can also be due to choice of leisure activities, such as watching TV or playing computer games.
- An sedentary lifestyle can lead to health issues such as obesity, heart disease and depression.

Late adulthood (70-84 years) and later adulthood (85+ years)

Dementia

- Dementia is a *degenerative* condition.
- There are different types of dementia, including **Alzheimer's**.
- Alzheimer's is caused by a build up of proteins in the brain which stops the normal functioning of nerve cells (neurones). This causes nerve cells to die, which disrupts brain functions.
- Symptoms of dementia include memory problems, mood swings and a reduced ability to carry out complex tasks.

Heart disease

Also known as **cardiovascular disease** this affects the heart, blood vessels and arteries.

- The heart's blood supply is disrupted or blocked by a build up of plaque in the coronary arteries. A build up of plaque in an artery is known as *atherosclerosis*.
- Symptoms of plaque in the coronary arteries include *angina*, shortness of breath and pain in the chest.
- If heart disease remains untreated it can result in a heart attack or heart failure.

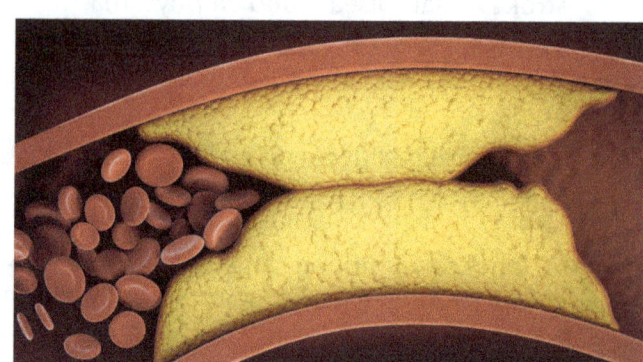

Oral health

- Natural wear and tear of teeth and gums leads to an increased risk of infections, inflammations, tooth decay/loss and dentures.
- Oral health conditions can also be caused by:
  » poor oral hygiene
  » some types of medications which cause a dry mouth. This removes saliva which helps protect teeth and gums from acids.

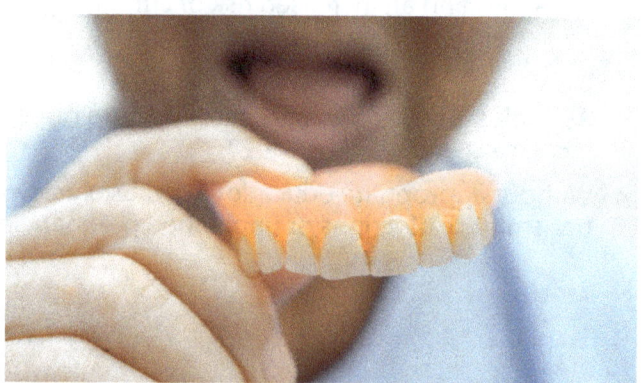

Injury from falls

- Older adults lose muscle mass, strength, balance and coordination. This all leads to an increased risk of falling.
- Conditions such as *osteoporosis* mean that a fall has more severe consequences due to weakened bones.
- Environmental conditions can also contribute to fall risks such as slippery surfaces or poor lighting.
- For these reasons hip fractures are common, and are very serious - 20-30% of people in the UK die within a year of a hip fracture because of further complications.
- A fall can pose further health risks such as broken bones or fractures, head traumas and cuts.

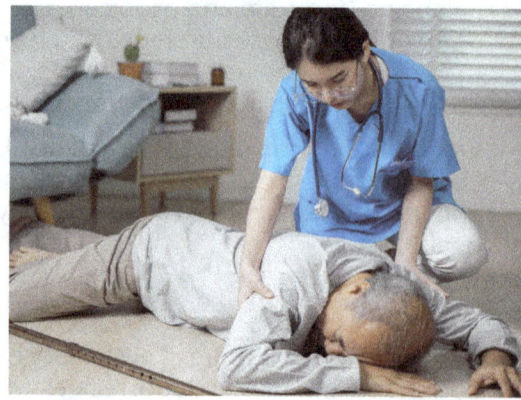

Weakened immune system

It is natural for the immune system to weaken with age. It is known as *immunosenescence*.

- The body's ability to fight off illness and infection is compromised, which can lead to further health complications.

- Elderly individuals have an increased risk of contracting influenza (flu) which can lead to further health issues such as ear infections and *pneumonia*.

Obesity

- Obesity is defined as a **body mass index (BMI)** of 30 or more.
- Develops when a large amount of excess fat is stored in the body. It can occur in any life stage.
- Can occur due to lack of exercise, poor lifestyle choices, poor diet, or due to genetic or medical conditions.
- Obesity is associated with a number of health problems, including poor mobility, type 2 diabetes, hypertension, cardiovascular disease and a number of types of cancer.

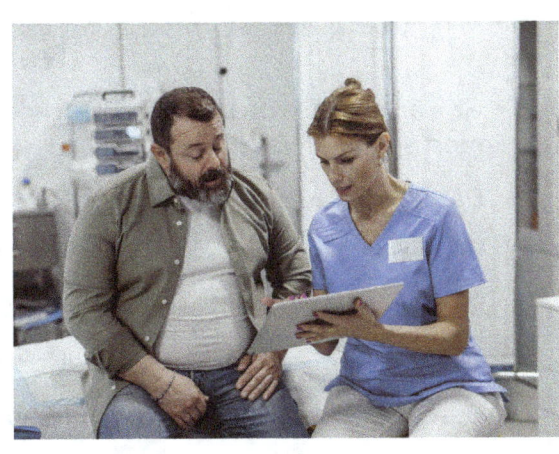

Study Tips!
- You need to be able to identify and understand specific health conditions relating to each life stage.
- Please note that although these conditions are specific to a life stage, some health conditions can occur across the life stages.
- You also need to be able to consider the effect of obesity in different life stages.

Important terms!

Contagious – when a health condition can be passed on to another person.

Bacterial – a condition that is caused by bacteria.

Viral – a condition caused by a virus.

Lethargy – a feeling of a lack of energy.

Inflammation – the body's response to an injury or infection and is seen through redness, soreness or swelling.

Nausea – a feeling of sickness.

Seizures – abnormal electrical activity in the brain causing unusual feelings or movements, including stiffness, twitching or convulsions.

Cirrhosis – scarring of the liver tissue that prevents the liver from functioning normally.

Degenerative – describes a condition that will get worse over time.

Amnesia – memory loss.

Atherosclerosis – a build up of plaque in the arteries, causing them to narrow and reduce blood flow. Can lead to heart attacks and strokes.

Angina – a condition that causes chest pain because the heart is not receiving enough oxygenated blood.

Osteoporosis – a condition that causes bones to lose density and strength.

Immunosenescence – the weakening of the immune system as part of the natural ageing process.

Pneumonia – inflammation of the lungs normally caused by a bacterial or viral infection. It can cause serious illness.

Recap Questions

1. Identify a prevalent health condition in infancy.
2. Identify a risk-taking behaviour in adolescence.
3. Give an example of a health issue relating to obesity.
4. How might an individual in middle adulthood acquire a brain injury?
5. What causes dental caries in early childhood?
6. What is heart disease?
7. Why do people in late and later adulthood have a weakened immune system?
8. Which health condition in infancy/early childhood is characterised by redness and secretions around the eyes?
9. In which life stages are depression and anxiety at work more likely?
10. Identify a factor that can contribute to a risk of injury via falling.

Revision Quiz

1. Give an example of an NHS health check. What age ranges might your chosen health check be most suitable for/
2. Describe the role of a psychiatrist.
3. What are Roper and Tierney's Activities of Daily Living and why are they used?
4. Describe two intellectual developments in infancy.
5. Why are multi-agency and multi-disciplinary approaches important in person-centred care?
6. Describe risk factors for health conditions that dentists commonly treat.
7. What is the role of a podiatrist?

C2 Health and social care promotion and prevention

Vaccinations

Vaccines are a type of medicine that teaches the body to create antibodies for a specific disease, so they become immune to that disease.

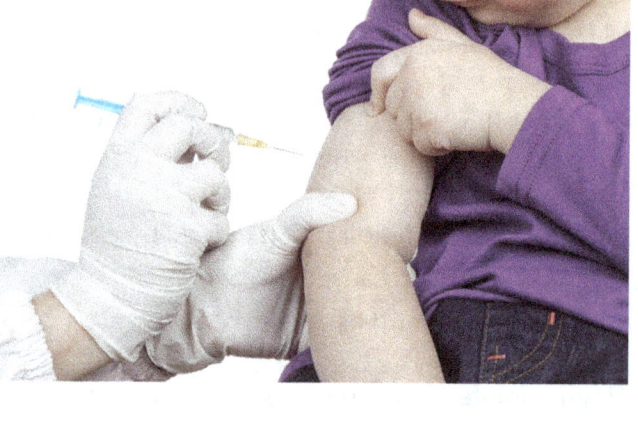

- They protect vulnerable individuals from potentially dangerous diseases.
- **Herd immunity** is when a large percentage of a population is immune to a disease. This protects the people who are not immune, because the disease cannot spread. Vaccines play an important role in herd immunity.

Vaccines can be given from the age of 8 weeks old into later adulthood.

- Common vaccines cover measles, mumps and rubella (MMR), polio, hepatitis B, tetanus, diphtheria, HPV and flu.
- There is a lot of misinformation about vaccines online. But vaccines have saved millions of lives.

Age-related health checks and screening

Checks and screening are used to discover if someone has a specific health issues or if they are at an increased risk of developing it due to genetic predisposition.

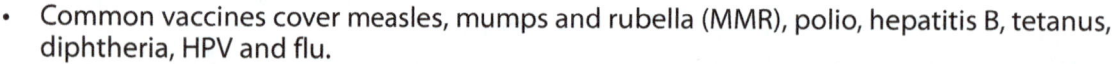

Checks and screening allow for healthcare professionals to provide an appropriate form of intervention.

Newborns

Hearing screening identifies any hearing loss or impairment.

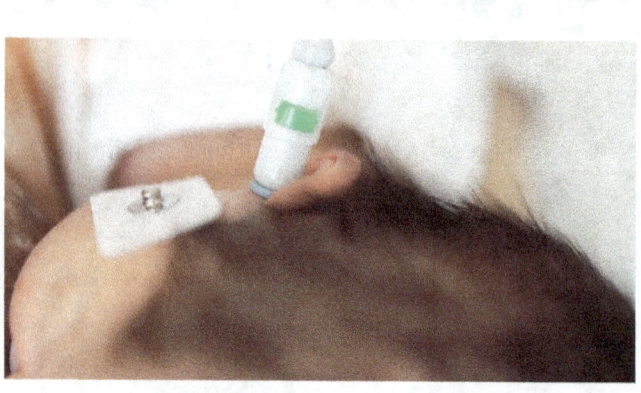

- The test is known as the **automated otoacoustic emission (AOAE)**.
- Soft earpieces placed in the ears play a clicking sound to see if there any hearing issues.

Infants

Health visitors continue to monitor and review **growth and development** of infants up until the age of 2 years.

- A **personal child health record (PCHR)** is completed by the health visitor so they can keep track of the infant's progression.
- It records height, weight and developmental milestones.
- Allows for any developmental delays to be identified early so that interventions can be put in place.

Hearing and eyesight checks

Hearing and eyesight checks are to determine any hearing or vision loss/impairment.

- Can be conducted at any life stage.
- The NHS targets individuals under 16, 60+ and those diagnosed with specific health conditions such as diabetes.

NHS health checks

The NHS offer a variety of health checks. These can be offered to at-risk individuals or to the general population who are over a certain age.

- **Diabetes checks** involve blood tests and blood sugar checks.
- **Hypertension** (high blood pressure) is reviewed using a sphygmomanometer.
- **Height and weight** are used to calculate body mass index (BMI) which is used to define obesity.
- **Cholesterol** checks involve blood tests and are used to check if someone is at risk of atherosclerosis.

Early cancer screening

- **Cervical cancer screening** ('smear test') is available for 25 to 64-year-olds, offered every three years.
- **Bowel cancer screening** is offered to everyone between the ages of 54–74.
- **Breast cancer screenings** (mammograms) are offered to people between the ages of 50–71 or younger people who are at greater risk of breast cancer

Dementia screening

- Dementia screening consists of **cognitive assessments** that test memory and thinking, **blood tests** and **brain scans**.
- There is no standard screen process in the UK but a GP can order the test if they suspect a patient has dementia.

Mental health education

Mental health education has raised awareness around different mental health conditions and their symptoms.

- Enables people to recognise the signs and symptoms of common conditions and seek help.
- Empowers individuals to make positive choices relating to their mental health.
- Reduces stigma around mental health and encourages open conversations about mental health and differing coping methods.

Education campaigns include national campaigns such as Every Mind Matters and Mental Health Awareness Week, leaflets and resources in public spaces, and coverage in the media.

Dental checks

- Annual dental checks are recommended for everyone. They can identify tooth decay, gum disease and other problems early, and recommend treatment to stop conditions getting worse.
- Dental checks are also part of wider oral health education, to encourage people to make healthy lifestyle choices for their gums and teeth.

Health education

Education about the health impacts of smoking, alcohol, drugs and sexual behaviour are important to help people make healthy lifestyle choices.

- Health education in schools encourages healthy behaviour at an early age.
- Promotes healthier communities by supporting individuals to make healthier informed decisions.
- Examples of health education campaigns include: Stoptober (smoking), Dry January (alcohol) and Sexual Health Week.

Accident prevention

Accidents cause many deaths and injuries each year. For example, around **1600 people are killed** in car accidents each year in the UK.

Accident prevention campaigns aim to change people's behaviour and attitudes to reduce preventable accidents. For example:

- **Road Safety Week** aims to involve schools and communities in road safety education.
- There have been numerous national campaigns to stop people from drink-driving and speeding.
- **Child Safety Week** highlights the hazards that children can face in the home, such as the risk of choking, poisoning and burns.

Study Tips!

- The health checks outlined are named on the specification, you can use your knowledge of other health checks as well.

Important terms!

Antibodies – proteins in the body that kill harmful bacteria and viruses.

Genetic predisposition – an increased chance of developing a condition because it runs in the family.

Health visitor – a professional that has a responsibility of supporting new parents and their babies.

Empowers – providing individuals with the opportunities to make their own choices or decisions.

Stigma – a prejudicial view individuals may have about certain individuals or health conditions.

Recap Questions

1. Define the term 'herd immunity'.
2. Give an example of a disease for which there is a vaccine.
3. Identify one health screening test conducted on newborns.
4. How are people educated about sexual health?
5. How is diabetes tested?
6. Why is mental health education important?
7. Identify a type of cancer that an individual can be screened for.
8. What does dental health education prevent?
9. Identify one accident prevention campaign.
10. Apart from diabetes, name one other NHS health check.

Revision Quiz

1. Outline the main features of Huntington's disease.
2. Describe the physical changes that occur during puberty.
3. What is 'synaptic pruning'?
4. Why might a person's social life improve in late adulthood? Why might it get worse?
5. Describe the positive impacts a healthy diet has on health.
6. What are the health impacts of drinking alcohol?
7. What impacts do environmental inequalities have on health?
8. Describe the links between discrimination and health outcomes.

C3 Health and social care professionals

Nurses

- **Mental health nurse** – role is to support recovery to encourage individuals to return to independent living.
  - » Work in settings such as psychiatry units, community healthcare centres, day care settings, residential settings and prisons.

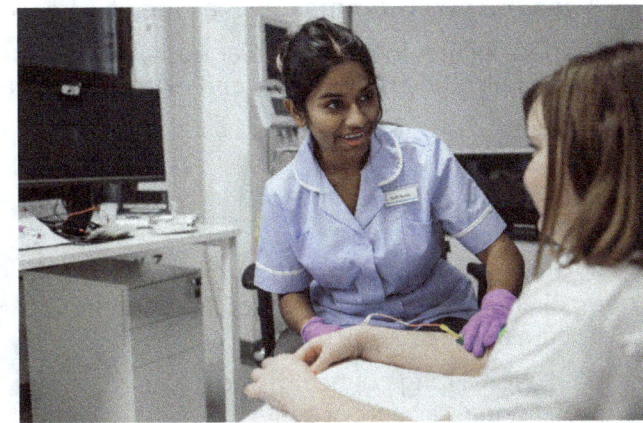

- **Adult nurse** – role is to support recovery by assessing and monitoring patients, administering medication, assisting with daily activities and completing administrative tasks.
  - » Work in settings such as hospitals, GP surgeries and can be part of domiciliary teams.
- **Learning disability nurse** – role is to support patients to be as independent as possible.
  - » Only work with individuals with learning disabilities.
  - » Work in community settings such as schools, in their own home or at work.
- **Children and young people (CYP) nurse** – support both the physical and emotional health of the child and family.
  - » Work in specific settings with designated paediatric wards.

Specialist community public health nurse – role is to support health outcomes and reduce health inequalities across communities. They include the following:

- **Health visitor** – role is to carry out regular assessment and reviews on the growth and development of infants to ensure developmental milestones are met and to provide early intervention if not.
  - » They work alongside other professionals to support infant development and often work in the patients' homes.
- **Children's practice nurse** – work specifically with children and are responsible for conducting health checks, taking blood samples, health screening and vaccinations.
  - » Work in GP surgeries.
- **School nurse (SN)** – employed directly in a school through the NHS.
  - » They are responsible for conducting vaccination programmes, health assessments, monitoring and reviewing health development and progression, identifying any potentially vulnerable children, supporting those with complex needs and promoting health education.
- **Occupational health nurse (OHN)** – based in the workplace, they conduct health needs assessments, provide health education to prevent accident and injury, and promote positive physical and mental health practices.

Midwives

- Provides care and support to women throughout pregnancy, childbirth and the postpartum period.
- Provide both antenatal and postnatal care.
- Support patients by monitoring mother and baby, providing health education for parents and children, helping to create birthing plans, aid in labour and delivery and provide emotional/mental health support.
- Based in a hospital's maternity unit or antenatal clinic, GP surgery and in patient's home.

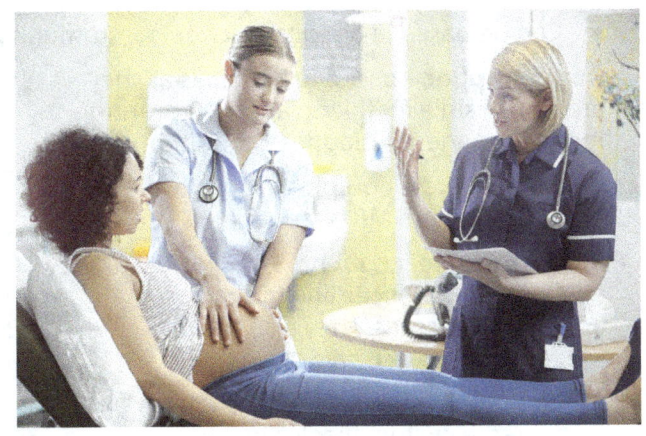

Doctors

General practitioner

- A **general practitioners** (GP) is a type of primary care professional.
- Responsibilities include the diagnosis, monitoring and reviewing of conditions, long-term patient care, prescribing medication, and referring patients to other professionals.

Surgeon

- **Surgeons** are an example of a tertiary care professional.
- Responsible for performing surgery to repair, remove or treat diseases, infections or damaged tissue/organs.
- Work with a range of healthcare professionals as part of a multi-disciplinary team.
- Example of surgeon speciality include neurosurgeon, cardiothoracic surgeon and trauma surgeon.

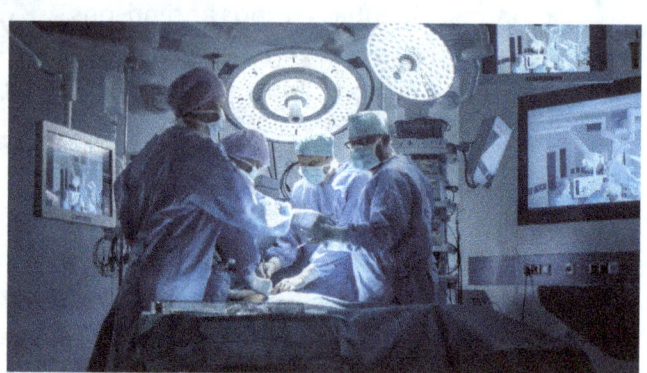

Psychiatrist

- A **psychiatrist** is a type of doctor responsible for diagnosing, treating and preventing mental health disorders.
- Conducts psychological evaluations of patients to determine severity of mental ill health.
- Works with a range of healthcare professionals to support the holistic needs of patients.
- Prescribes medicine or talking therapies to help people with mental health conditions.

Allied professions

- **Physiotherapist** – supports patients with physical issues that impact mobility.
  » They offer treatments such as massage therapy or exercises.
- **Occupational therapist** – supports patients of all ages that struggle with day-to-day tasks.
  » They will assess an individual's capabilities and then suggest adjustments to the home or activities in order to promote independence.

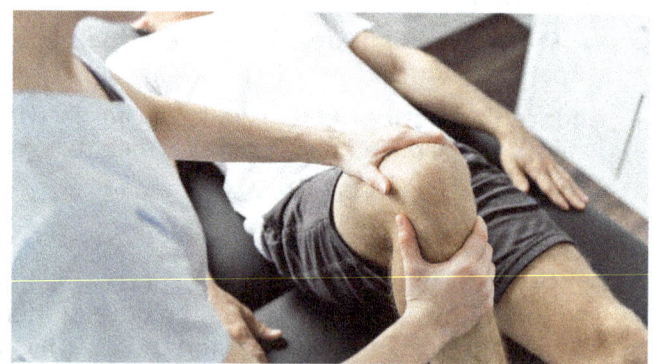

- **Speech therapist** – assesses and treats issues with speech, language, swallowing and communication.
  » Can be based in hospitals, schools, community health centres, prisons and day centres.
- **Radiographer** – based in hospitals as they are responsible for taking and interpreting medical images to diagnose conditions.
  » They operate equipment such as X-ray machines and MRI scanners.
- **Podiatrist** – treat patients with foot or ankle problems, including infections and mobility issues. They also provide preventative advice and care.
  » Can provide patients with exercises or create custom insoles for shoes to maintain movement.

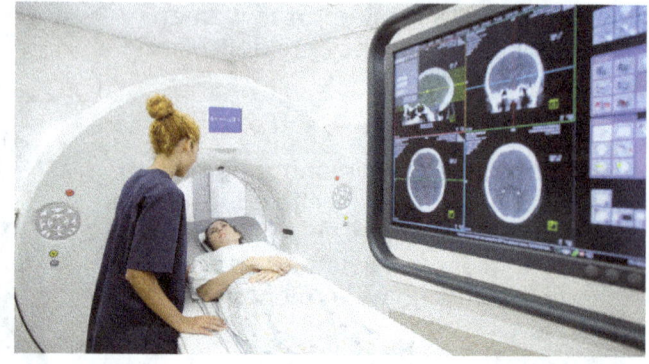

Dental care

Dentists are primary care professionals responsible for monitoring and maintaining the oral health of the community they work in.

- Monitor oral health through regular check-ups.
- Provide treatments such as fillings, root canal treatment, dentures and cosmetic treatments.
- Also play an important role in the health education of their local community.

Dental hygienists provide preventative care for patients that have been referred to them by a dentist.

- They also educate patients on how to maintain good oral hygiene through brushing teeth.

Social worker

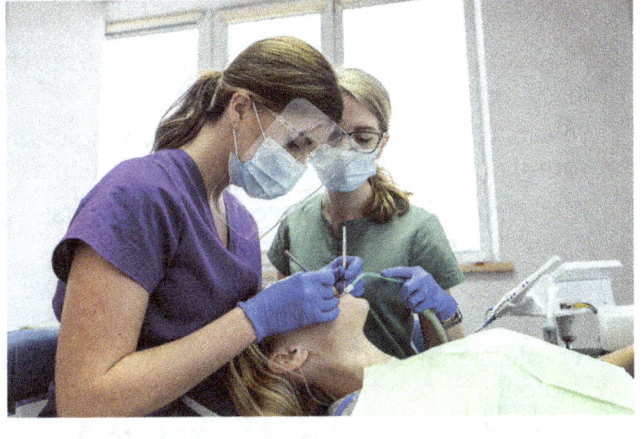

- **Social workers** support individuals with a variety of social problems.
- They specialise in working with children and young people or adults.
- Primary aim is to protect vulnerable people from harm and to improve people's lives.
- They are responsible for assessing the circumstances of individuals to determine the support and help they might need, including from a range of other professionals.
- Support a wide range of people including those with disabilities, those living in poverty, children in care, children or adults at risk of abuse, young offenders and children being fostered or adopted.

Dietician

Responsible for supporting issues around diet and nutrition, including obesity and malnutrition.

- They design and implement nutrition plans and provide information and advice about diet and foods to empower individuals.

Care and support workers

- They support people struggling with day-to-day living due to issues with age, illness, injury or disability.
- They also provide companionship and emotional support.
- When providing personal care, they must ensure the dignity of the patient is maintained.
- There are domiciliary carers (who visit people at their homes) and residential carers (for those in care homes).

Psychologist and counsellor

A **psychologist** is not a medical doctor an cannot prescribe medicine. However they require advanced degrees in psychology to be able to practice in the UK.

» They support people with mental health conditions such as depression and schizophrenia.

A **counsellor** can support a wider range of issues such as bereavement and relationship difficulties.

- Both psychologists and counsellors may opt to use talking therapies to support individuals and provide them with coping methods, so they are better able to support themselves.

Youth worker

- They support and mentor young people from the ages of 11-19, and those with additional needs up to the age of 25.
- They act as trusted adults who help young people develop and reach their potential. They help young people with a range of life skills, such as how to complete a job application.
- They also collaborate with other professionals, such as social workers, teachers and people running community groups.

Social prescriber

- A professional that refers people to non-clinical services to help improve people's health and wellbeing.
- The fundamental idea is that some people visit services such as GPs with non-medical problems, which takes up resources and does not necessarily help them. Social prescribers try to understand the non-clinical issues that people might have, focusing on *holistic* health and wellbeing.
- Social prescribers have begun to be integrated into primary care services, so that individuals have access to a variety of resources and services to suit their needs.

> **Study Tips!**
> - You need to be able to link appropriate professionals to the conditions described in C1.
> - You need to understand and be able to describe the role of each professional.

C4 Personalised care and multi-disciplinary working

Integrated care systems

- Allows different services to form a partnership to ensure individuals receive high quality care.
- An ICS requires all services and professionals to take a similar approach to care and maintain a high level of communication with each other.
- Requires a multi-disciplinary approach: which is when different professionals from the same service work together e.g. a physiotherapist and a doctor in a hospital.
- Also requires a *multi-agency* approach: which is when professionals from different services work together e.g. a health visitor and a social worker.

Person-centred approach to care

This approach considers the holistic needs of an individual.

- Professionals will first assess the individual to determine the needs that require support.
- **Roper and Tierney** created a model called the **Activities of Daily Living** for this assessment. It considers how an individual's life has been impacted by an illness or injury.
- The model considers activities needed for daily living such as eating, being mobile and sleeping.

Features of multi-disciplinary team working

- **Shared decision making** – all professionals involved in the care and treatment of a service user should be informed of all decisions made. Professionals should have the opportunity to discuss the decisions first, in order to make an informed decision.
- **Professionals working together** – multi-disciplinary and multi-agency teams must:
  - » Establish and agree upon effective ways of working and communicating. This ensure all the professionals are fully involved and know what is happening. This is vital in order to provide high quality care.
  - » Understand each other's roles, in order to appreciate the challenges and constraints that they all face, and the positive impacts they can have on the service user.
- **Working with families and significant others** – those closest to the patient should be kept informed of all decisions made by and with professionals. A nominated professional should be the main source of communication with the patient's family.

Study Tips!
- You need to be able to identify and outline the relevant professionals that could support an individual based on your knowledge from C3 content.
- You need to be able to explain the purpose of multi-disciplinary teams.

Important terms!

Domiciliary teams – professionals that support patients in their own home.

Paediatric wards – a department of a hospital providing care to children.

Postpartum period – the weeks after childbirth.

Antenatal care – care and support provided whilst the woman is pregnant.

Postnatal care – care and support provided to mother and baby after birth.

Primary care – the first place an individual can go to for healthcare support.

Tertiary care – specialised professionals/services who primary care patients are referred to.

Multi-disciplinary team – when a group of professionals from a range of specialisms work together to support a patient.

Neurosurgeon – a surgeon that specialises in the brain and nervous system.

Cardiothoracic surgeon – a surgeon that operates on the heart, lungs and vital chest organs.

Holistic – considering all of an individual's needs not just the physical.

Malnutrition – not consuming the right amount and type of nutrients.

Personal care – intimate care including washing, toileting and dressing.

Dignity – how worthy a person feels, based on the care provided.

Residential carer – a care or support worker based in a setting such as a care home.

Bereavement – the death of a loved one.

Multi-agency – different teams from differing services work together to support one patient.

Recap Questions

1. Identify a professional that supports individuals with their diet.
2. Name two types of nurses.
3. Name a type of doctor that works in primary care.
4. Outline the role of a midwife.
5. Identify two types of allied health professional.
6. What is the main purpose of a dentist?
7. Which type of professional is most appropriate for supporting an individual with schizophrenia?
8. What is a social prescriber?
9. Identify two life stages a youth worker is more likely to support.
10. Define the term 'domiciliary'.
11. What is an integrated care system?
12. What is a person-centred approach?
13. Define the term 'holistic'.
14. Who developed a model that considers activities of daily living?
15. Why is communication between all those involved a multi-disciplinary team important?
16. Apart from professionals, who else do multi-disciplinary teams need to work with?
17. Identify a daily activity that might be considered when assessing the needs of an individual for person-centred care.
18. Why is it important for professionals to share decisions?
19. What is the difference between a multi-disciplinary team and a multi-agency team?
20. What are the possible implications of a multi-disciplinary team failing?

Revision Quiz

1. What is a common health condition in late adulthood?
2. What are the impacts of substance misuse in adolescents?
3. Describe the main features of cystic fibrosis.
4. What are the risk factors for developing prostate cancer?
5. What happens to the joints and bones in later adulthood?
6. What age range is the definition of middle adulthood? Why my libido be affected in this age range?
7. What are three symptoms of menopause?
8. At what age range does emotional regulation begin to develop?

Assessment practice

1. Identify which healthcare professional can help an individual with teeth brushing techniques. (1)
2. Identify a prevalent health condition in late adulthood. (1)
3. Describe the concept of herd immunity. (1)
4. State the branch of nursing concerned with supporting new mothers and their babies. (1)
5. Explain two ways a midwife and a social worker can work together to support an individual living in poverty. (4)
6. Give one setting other than a hospital where a psychiatrist may work. (1)
7. State the definition of a multi-disciplinary team. (1)
8. Identify two features of multi-disciplinary team working. (2)
9. Explain the main purpose of vaccinations. (2)
10. Identify a health check that an individual in middle adulthood might need. (1)
11. Explain one reason for obesity in adolescence. (2)
12. Evaluate the role of a youth worker when working with an individual to improve their diet. (9)

Unit 2 Human biology and health

A Organisation of the human body

The **cell** is the basic unit of life.

- Billions of cells work together to form **tissues**. Tissues are specialised groups of cells with a common function.
- Tissues combine to create **organs**, which carry out specific tasks in the body, and organs work together to form organ systems.

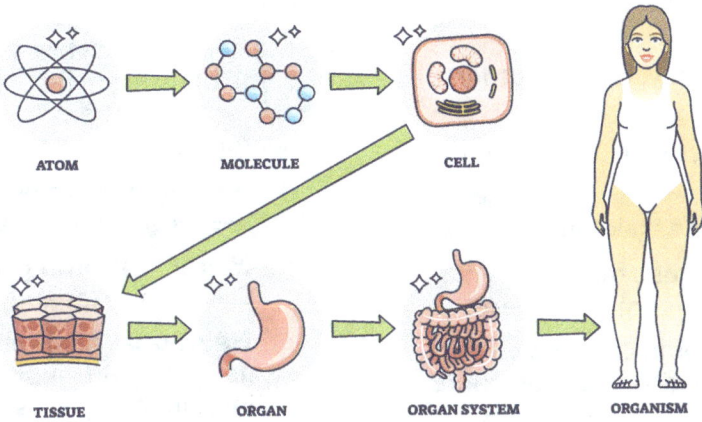

A1 Cells

Cells are the basic building block of life. They make up all living organisms. The average adult has approximately 32 trillion cells in their body.

Nucleus
- The 'control centre' of the cell.
- Surrounded by a membrane, and contains the cell's genetic material, DNA.

Ribosomes
- The smallest of the cell organelles.
- They produce proteins (**protein synthesis**).

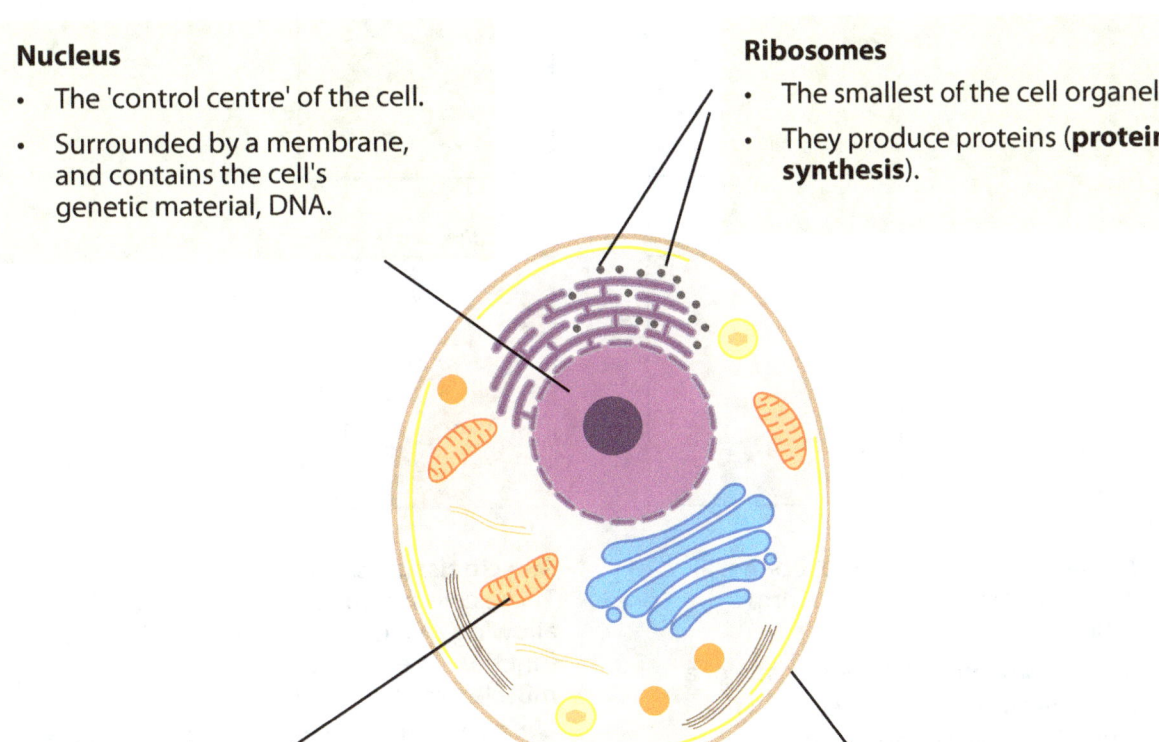

Mitochondria
- The 'powerhouses' of the cell.
- They release energy that can be used by the cell.
- Mitochondria contain **enzymes** that perform the process of cellular respiration.

Cell membrane
- Forms a flexible barrier.
- **Selectively permeable** – allows substances like oxygen and glucose to enter the cell, and waste products like CO_2 to leave the cell

A2 Tissues

Connective tissue is like the scaffolding of your body. It holds everything together, provides support, protection, and insulation and connects the different systems of the body.

There are several different types of connective tissue:

- **Blood** – transports oxygen and nutrients around the body.
- **Cartilage** – provides structure, support and cushioning.
- **Bone** – makes up the skeleton.
- **Areolar tissue** – forms a mesh-like structure which holds organs in place.
- **Adipose tissue** – commonly known as fat, it provides insulation and protection.

Nervous tissue is the specialised tissue that makes up the brain, spinal cord, and nerves. It is responsible for receiving, processing, and transmitting information throughout the body.

- The brain and spinal cord form the central nervous system (CNS).
- The nerves which branch out to every part of the body form the peripheral nervous system (PNS). There are different types of neurones:
  » **Sensory neurones** transmit signals from the sensory receptors to the CNS.
  » **Motor neurones** carry signals from the CNS to muscles and glands.
  » **Neuroglia (glial cells)** provide the other neurones with support, protection and insulation (myelin sheaths).

Connective tissue

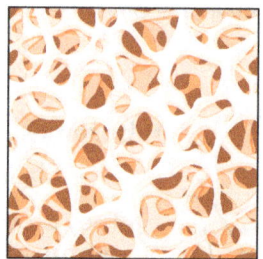

Neural tissue

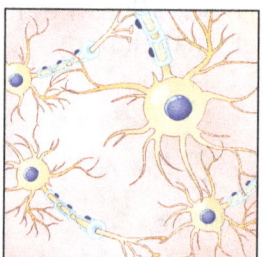

Epithelial tissue

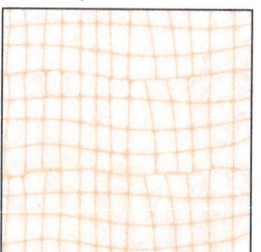

Muscle tissue

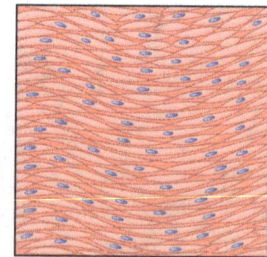

Epithelial tissue is made up of epithelial cells tightly packed together to form a continuous sheet.

- **Simple epithelial tissue** is made of a single layer of cells. It is found in the alveoli and blood capillaries.
- **Compound epithelial tissue** is made up of multiple layers of cells. It is tougher and provides more protection. It is found in places that experience a lot of wear and tear, like your skin.
- Epithelial tissue has several important jobs: protection, absorption, excretion, filtration and sensory reception.

Muscle tissue is made up of muscle cells. These cells are specialised for contraction, allowing movement, posture, and organ function. There are three main types of muscle tissue:

- **Striated** (skeletal) – attached to bones by tendons. It is under voluntary control and is responsible for movement.
- **Non-striated** (smooth) – found in the walls of internal organs like the digestive system. It is not under voluntary control.
- **Cardiac** – only found in the heart. It is not under voluntary control, to ensure the heart pumps blood continuously.

A3 Energy in the body

Energy metabolism

Metabolism is made up of two processes: **catabolism** and **anabolism**.

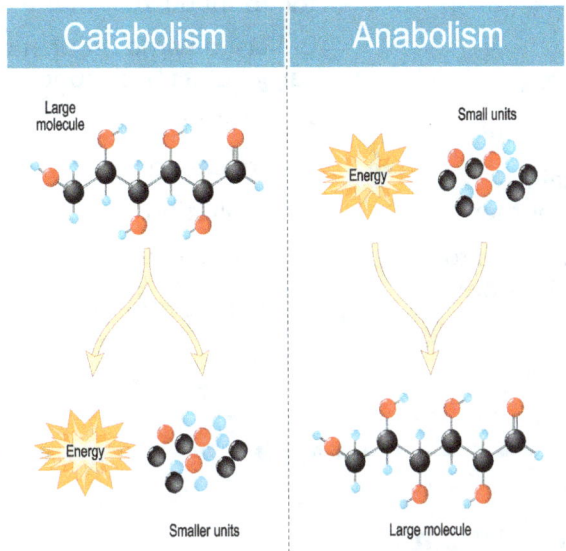

Catabolism: the process of **breaking down complex molecules** into simpler ones to release energy. This energy is used for all the body's functions, from muscle movement to brain activity.

Nutrients like **carbohydrates**, **proteins**, and **fats** get broken down during catabolism.

Anabolism: uses energy to **build complex molecules** from simpler ones.

Anabolism is how our bodies create proteins, carbohydrates, lipids, and **nucleic acids**, which are the building blocks of life.

Cellular Respiration

Aerobic respiration is the process by which cells convert glucose into energy **in the presence of oxygen**.

It involves a series of chemical reactions which breaks down glucose step by step.

Along the way, energy is released and captured in the form of ATP, the energy currency of the cell.

This process occurs in several stages:

- **Stage 1** occurs in the **cytoplasm**. Glucose is partially broken down producing a small amount of ATP. The broken-down glucose is then transported into the mitochondria.

- **Stage 2** happens inside the **mitochondria**. A series of reactions finishes breaking down the glucose. This releases carbon dioxide. Oxygen is used up and water is produced. This generates a large amount of ATP.

The reaction can be summarised by the equation:

$$\text{glucose} + \text{oxygen} \rightarrow \text{carbon dioxide} + \text{water} + \text{ATP}$$

Anaerobic respiration is the process of producing ATP **without the presence of oxygen**:

- Occurs in the **cytoplasm**.
- Much less efficient way to produce ATP compared to aerobic respiration.
- Takes place when oxygen levels are low or absent.
- Produces **lactic acid** as the end product, which can quickly cause muscle fatigue.
- Only produces a small amount of ATP, and quickly leads to a buildup of lactic acid.

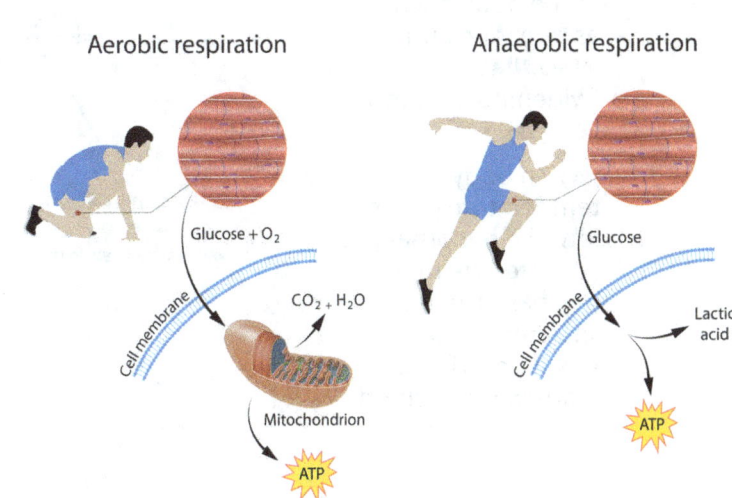

Uses of energy in the body

Energy is used for the following processes:

- Cell division for growth and repair.
- Passage of nerve impulses.
- Contraction of muscle tissue.
- Homeostasis to maintain a constant internal environment.
- Anabolism: Energy is needed to build complex molecules from simpler ones.

Basal Metabolic Rate (**BMR**) is the amount of energy your body burns while at complete rest. It accounts for about 60-70% of the calories we use each day.

BMR is the amount of energy your body needs to carry out its basic functions like:

- breathing
- circulating blood
- respiration
- maintaining body temperature
- keeping your organs functioning.

A4 Homeostatic mechanisms

Homeostasis is defined as 'the ability of the body to maintain a stable internal environment despite changes in external conditions'.

Our bodies constantly monitor and regulate a range of factors, such as temperature, fluid balance, and sugar levels, to ensure optimal conditions for cells and organs to function properly. Our bodies use **negative feedback loops** to maintain this equilibrium.

Thermoregulation uses negative feedback to maintain a stable internal temperature:

- When body temperature goes above or below the normal range, temperature sensors in the skin and brain send information to the **hypothalamus** (in the brain).
  - » When body temperature is too high, the hypothalamus responds by initiating cooling mechanisms in the body, such as sweating and **vasodilation** (widening of blood vessels).
  - » When body temperature is too low, the hypothalamus activates warming mechanisms like shivering and **vasoconstriction** (narrowing of blood vessels).

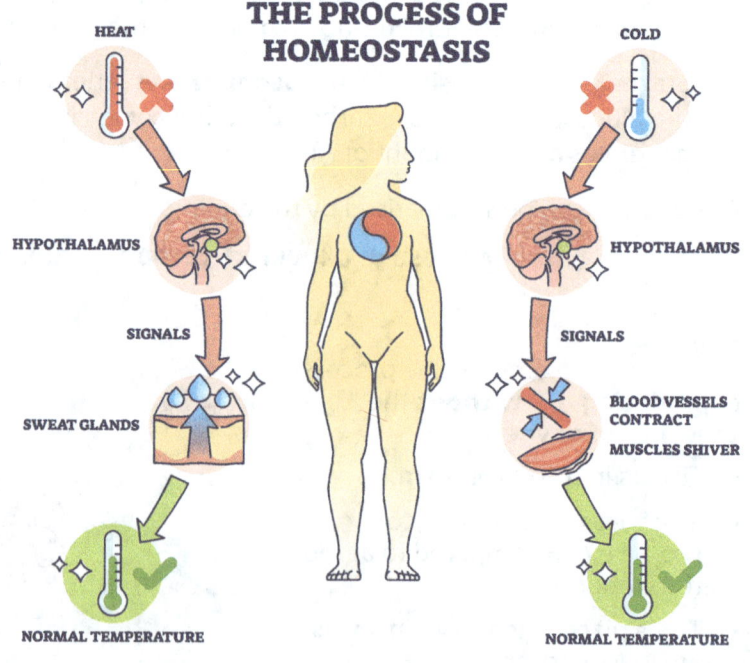

Glucoregulation means maintaining a steady blood sugar level.

- When blood sugar levels rise after eating, the pancreas releases **insulin**, a hormone which stimulates:
  » glucose uptake by cells
  » glucose storage as **glycogen** in the liver and muscles.
- Both of these reduce blood sugar levels back to normal.
- If blood sugar levels drop too low, the pancreas releases glucagon, which breaks down glycogen into glucose and releases it into the bloodstream.

The pancreas constantly monitors blood glucose levels throughout the day to ensure they stay within the correct range.

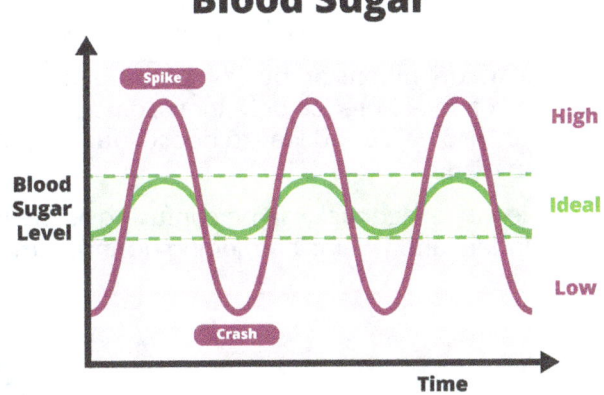

Osmoregulation is the body's process of maintaining the correct balance of water and salts in the body. Without it, cells could become either dehydrated or swollen, which could lead to organ failure.

Special receptors called **osmoreceptors** detect changes in blood solute concentration:

- If the body is dehydrated, the hypothalamus (in the brain) stimulates the release of **antidiuretic hormone** (**ADH**), which signals the kidneys to reabsorb more water.
- If the body is over-hydrated, ADH production decreases, resulting in increased water excretion.

This feedback loop ensures that the body's water content remains within a narrow range.

Important terms!

CNS – central nervous system. Made up of the brain and spinal cord.

PNS – peripheral nervous system. The nerves which branch out to every part of the body.

Catabolism – the process of breaking down complex molecules into simpler ones to release energy.

Anabolism – uses energy to build complex molecules from simpler ones.

Aerobic respiration – the process by which cells convert glucose into energy in the presence of oxygen.

Anaerobic respiration – the process by which cells convert glucose into energy **not** in the presence of oxygen.

ATP – the form of energy that the body's cells use.

BMR – the amount of energy your body burns while at complete rest. It accounts for about 60-70% of the calories we use each day.

Homeostasis – the ability of the body to maintain a stable internal environment despite changes in external conditions.

Thermoregulation – maintaining a stable body temperature.

Glucoregulation – maintaining a stable blood glucose level.

Osmoregulation – maintaining the correct balance of water and salts in the body.

Study Tips!

- Make sure you can use the scientific vocabulary correctly in your response – there are usually some marks available for using the specific words.
- Learn definitions off by heart. For example, the definition of homeostasis. Examiners often look for very precise definitions, particularly if they have been given in the specification. This can also be a good way to boost your confidence in the exam as it can be an easy way to pick up marks.
- Negative feedback can be confusing as the body is acting against the change. Take time to understand what is happening during homeostasis.

Recap Questions

1. What is the function of the cell membrane?
2. Which cell organelle is known as the 'control centre' and contains DNA?
3. What is the main function of mitochondria?
4. What are the four main types of tissue in the body?
5. What is the function of epithelial tissue?
6. Name three types of connective tissue.
7. What are the three types of muscle tissue?
8. What is the function of nervous tissue?
9. What is the process of breaking down complex molecules into simpler ones to release energy called?
10. What are the end products of aerobic respiration?
11. What is the end product of anaerobic respiration in muscles?
12. What is Basal Metabolic Rate (BMR)?
13. What is homeostasis?
14. What is the process of maintaining a stable internal body temperature called?
15. Which hormone is released by the pancreas when blood sugar levels are high?

Revision Quiz

1. Describe the pathway of blood through the heart, starting from the vena cava.
2. Name three hormones and their functions.
3. What are the differences between skeletal, smooth, and cardiac muscle?
4. What is a Transient Ischemic Attack (TIA)?
5. What are the main triggers of asthma?
6. How does obesity contribute to the development of type 2 diabetes?
7. What are some of the primary and secondary effects of dementia on communication and language skills?
8. What are the main risk factors associated with bowel cancer?
9. Describe the role of enzymes in digestion.

Assessment practice - Section A

1. Identify one type of connective tissue from the following list. (1)

    b) Neuroglia

    c) Striated

    d) Cartilage

    e) Sensory neurones

2. Label the parts of this cell. (4)

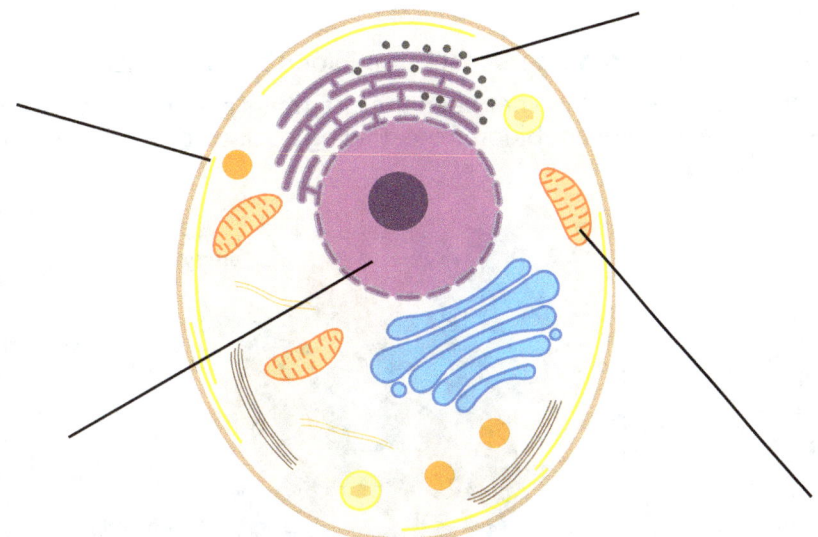

3. Describe the function of:

    b) Mitochondria

    c) Ribosomes. (2)

4. Explain the difference between anabolism and catabolism. (2)

5. Complete the word equation for aerobic respiration: (2)

    glucose + ……………………….. --> ………………………… + water

6. Describe the differences between aerobic and anaerobic respiration. (3)

7. State three ways energy is used in the body. (3)

8. State the definition of homeostasis. (1)

9. Describe the mechanisms used by the body to maintain a constant temperature. (5)

10. Circle the names of the two hormones involved in regulation of blood glucose. (2)

    glucagon   glycogen   insulin   ADH

11. Describe how the endocrine system regulates blood glucose levels (5)

12. Describe how the brain and the kidneys work together to maintain the correct balance of water in the body, and explain the importance of this. (5)

B Body systems

B1 The cardiovascular system

The heart is divided into four chambers:
- the right atrium
- the right ventricle
- the left atrium
- the left ventricle.

The **atria** are the **upper chambers** that receive blood being returned from the body,

The **ventricles** are the **lower chambers** that pump blood out of the heart.

Four valves control the flow of blood between the chambers and into and out of the heart. The valves prevent blood from flowing backward, ensuring a one-way flow of blood.

> **Study Tip!**
> Don't get the heart chambers muddled up – on diagrams the right atrium and right ventricle are shown on the left, and the left atrium and left ventricle are shown on the right!

The **right atrium** receives deoxygenated blood from the body through the superior and inferior **vena cava**. This blood is then pumped to the **right ventricle** and then to the lungs through the **pulmonary artery** to pick up oxygen.

The oxygenated blood then returns to the **left side of the heart** through the **pulmonary veins**.

From the **left atrium**, blood is pumped into the **left ventricle**, which then pumps it into the **aorta**, the body's largest artery.

This **oxygenated blood is then distributed throughout the body** through a network of arteries and capillaries.

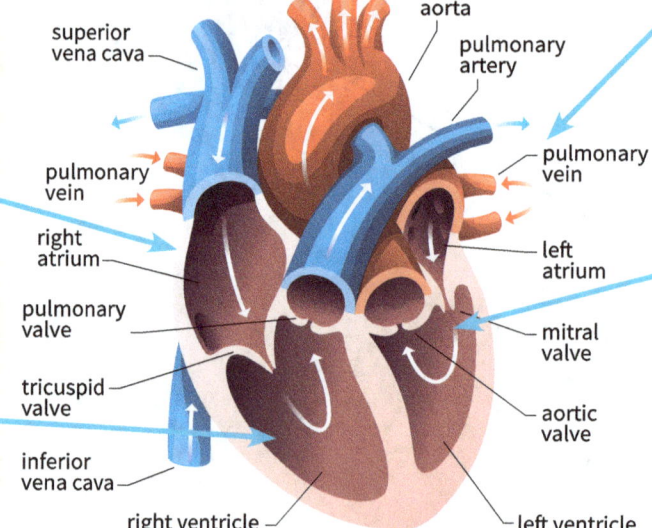

The circulatory system has two parts:
- The pulmonary circulatory system takes deoxygenated blood from the heart to the lungs and returns oxygenated blood back to the heart.
- The systemic circulatory system takes oxygenated blood from the heart and takes it around the body, returning deoxygenated blood to the heart.

Cardiac cycle

The cardiac cycle is the sequence of events that occur during one complete heartbeat.

Specialised muscle cells (cardiac muscle cells) in the heart, generate **electrical impulses** that cause the heart muscle to **contract in a coordinated rhythm**.

There are two main elements in the cycle:
- Systole – when the heart contracts and pumps blood out.
- Diastole – when the heart relaxes and fills with blood.

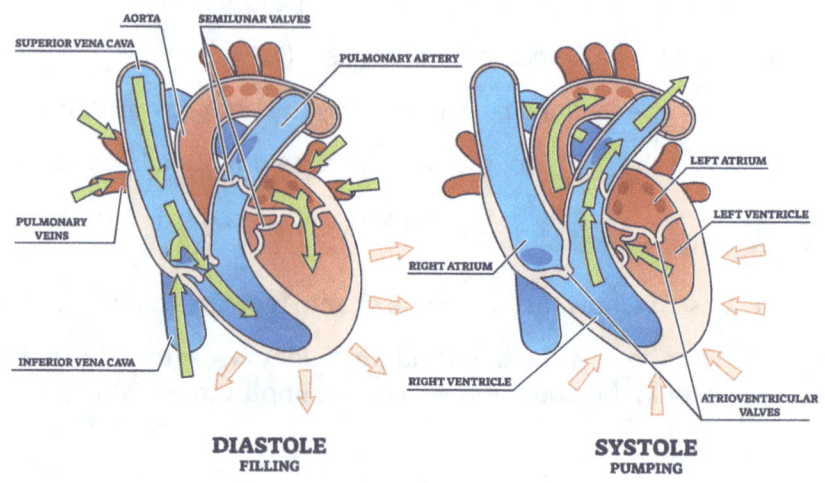

46

The cycle begins with atrial systole, where the atria contract, forcing blood into the ventricles. The ventricles are then filled with blood, and the atria relax.

Next comes ventricular systole, where the ventricles contract, pushing blood out of the heart into the arteries. The left ventricle pumps blood into the aorta, which carries oxygenated blood to the body. The right ventricle pumps blood into the pulmonary artery, which carries deoxygenated blood to the lungs.

Diastole is the brief period where the heart chambers relax and the atria fill with blood before the cycle starts again.

Structure of blood vessels

Blood vessels form a vast network that transports blood throughout the body. There are three main types: arteries, veins, and capillaries.

Arteries

- Arteries carry blood away from the heart.
- Have thick, muscular walls to withstand the high pressure of blood pumped by the heart. The largest artery is the aorta.
- As arteries branch into smaller vessels, they become arterioles, which eventually narrow into capillaries.

Veins

- Veins carry blood back to the heart.
- They have thinner walls than arteries.
- Contain valves to prevent blood from flowing backwards.
- Collect **deoxygenated** blood (blood that has low oxygen levels) from the body's tissues and return it to the right atrium of the heart.

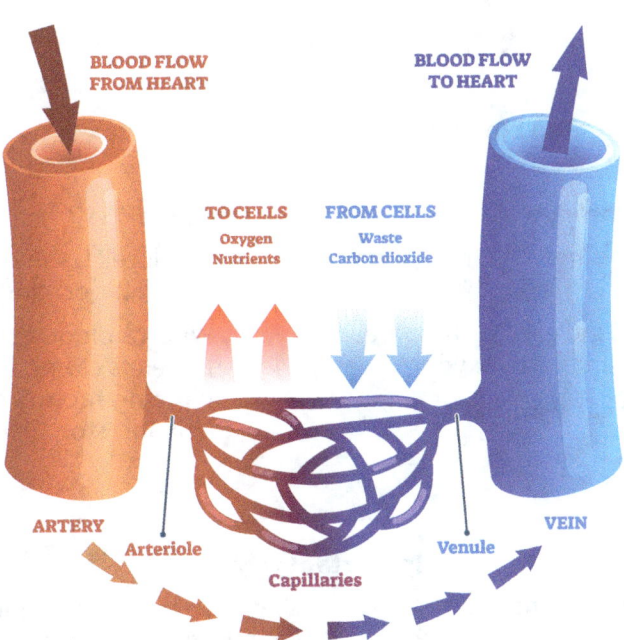

Capillaries

- Capillaries are the smallest blood vessels that form a network that reaches every cell in the body.
- They have very thin walls, which allows for the exchange of oxygen, nutrients, and waste products between the blood and the surrounding tissues.

Structure of blood

Blood is a tissue made up of several components, each with a specific function. These components include plasma, red blood cells, white blood cells, and platelets.

Plasma
- Liquid part of the blood.
- Makes up about 55% of its total volume.
- Mixture of water, proteins, ions, and other substances.
- Transports substances around the body.

White blood cells (leukocytes)
- Part of the immune system and help fight infection.
- There are different types each with a specific function.
- Some white blood cells engulf and destroy bacteria and other pathogens.
- Others produce antibodies to help neutralise pathogens.
- There are fewer white blood cells than red blood cells.

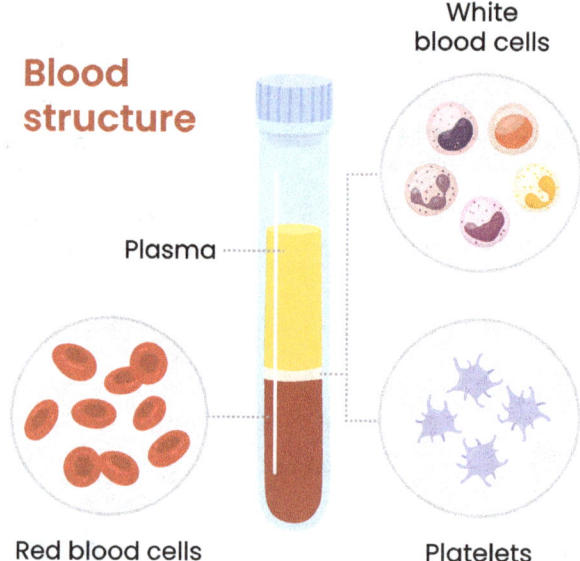

Blood structure

Red blood cells (erythrocytes)
- Contain **haemoglobin** which transports oxygen.
- Biconcave shape to increase surface area – allows increased uptake of oxygen.
- No nucleus, so can carry more haemoglobin.

Platelets
- Small cell fragments that play a crucial role in blood clotting.
- When a blood vessel is damaged, platelets clump together and release **clotting factors**, which help to form a clot and stop bleeding.

Important terms!

Deoxygenated blood – blood that doesn't contain much oxygen. Usually found in the veins.

Oxygenated blood – blood that contains lots of oxygen. Usually found in the arteries.

Atrial systole - when the atria contract, forcing blood into the ventricles.

Ventricular systole - when the ventricles contract, pushing blood out of the heart into the arteries.

Diastole - the brief period where the heart chambers relax and the atria fill with blood before the cardiac cycle starts again.

Arteries – thick-walled vessels that carry blood away from the heart.

Veins - vessels that carry blood back to the heart.

Capillaries - smallest blood vessels that form a network that reaches every cell in the body.

Haemoglobin – a substance found in red blood cells that carries oxygen.

B2 The respiratory system

Structure and function of the trachea and lungs

The respiratory system consists of the:
- trachea
- lungs
- bronchi
- bronchioles
- alveoli

Trachea (windpipe)
- A tube that connects the larynx (voice box) to the bronchi, the passageways leading to the lungs.
- Surrounded by rings of cartilage.
- Lined with a mucous membrane that produces mucus.
- **Ciliated cells** have hair-like structures (**cilia**) which move the mucus upwards, away from the lungs.

Lungs
- A pair of spongy organs located on either side of the chest.
- Enclosed by the ribcage and diaphragm, which help to expand and contract the lungs during breathing.

Bronchi
- The trachea divides into two **bronchi**, one leading to each lung.

Bronchioles
- The bronchi divide into smaller and smaller tubes called **bronchioles**.
- The bronchioles end in tiny air sacs called **alveoli**.

Alveoli
- Where **gas exchange** occurs.
- The walls of the alveoli are very thin.
- The alveoli are surrounded by capillaries, which carry blood to and from the lungs.
- Oxygen from the alveoli **diffuses** into the blood, while carbon dioxide from the blood diffuses into the alveoli to be exhaled.

Ventilation

Gas exchange

Gas exchange is the process by which oxygen is taken into the body and carbon dioxide is expelled.

Gas exchange occurs at the alveoli in the lungs.

- When you inhale, air travels through the trachea, bronchi, and bronchioles, eventually reaching the alveoli.
- Oxygen molecules diffuse across the thin walls of the alveoli and into the blood capillaries.
- Oxygen molecules then bind to **haemoglobin** in red blood cells, which transports the oxygen to the body's tissues.
- Carbon dioxide, a waste product of cellular respiration, diffuses from the blood capillaries into the alveoli. This carbon dioxide is then exhaled when you breathe out.

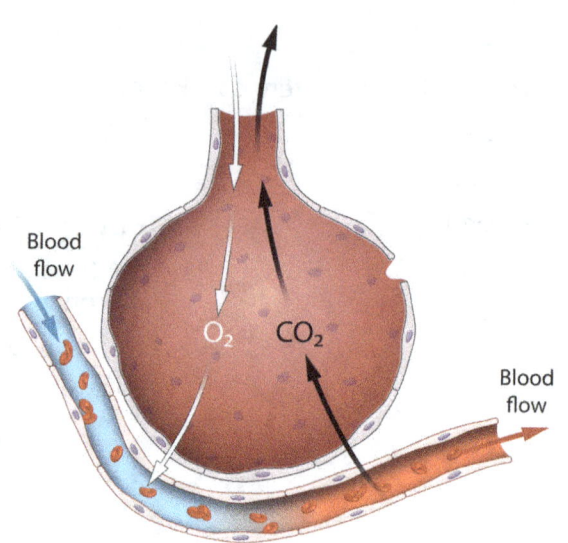

Diaphragm and intercostal muscles

The diaphragm and intercostal muscles are responsible for bringing about the process of breathing.

- The intercostal muscles are located between the ribs.
- The diaphragm is a dome-shaped muscle that separates the thorax (chest cavity) from the abdominal cavity. (The abdominal cavity is the space within the abdomen that contains the liver, pancreas, stomach and intestines.)

Inhaling

- The **diaphragm** contracts and flattens **downward**.
- The **intercostal muscles contract** lifting the ribcage upward and outward.
- This **increases the volume** of the thorax, which **decreases the pressure** inside the chest.
- This lower pressure pulls air into the lungs.

Exhaling

- The **diaphragm relaxes** and moves **upward**.
- The **intercostal muscles relax**, and the ribcage moves downwards and inwards.
- This **decreases the volume** of the thorax, which **increases the pressure** inside the thorax.
- The increased pressure pushes air out of the lungs.

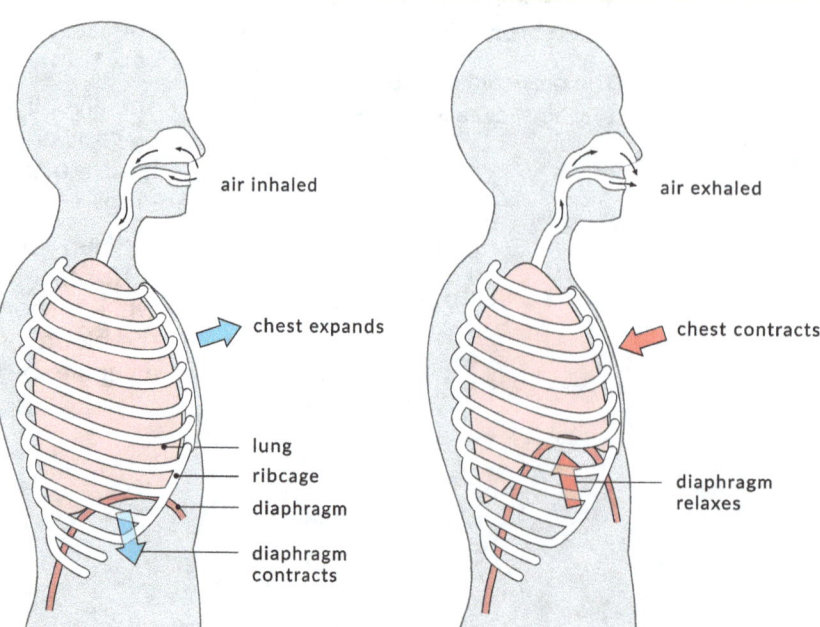

> **Study Tips!**
> It's important to be able to explain the movement of air into and out of the lungs in terms of pressure changes in the thorax.
>
> An **increase in volume** causes a **decrease in pressure** which pulls air into the lungs.

Important terms!

Gas exchange – where oxygen diffuses into the blood and carbon dioxide diffuses out of the blood.

Diffuse – the movement of molecules down a concentration gradient i.e. from an area of high concentration to an area of low concentration.

Alveoli – the tiny air sacs in the lungs where gas exchange occurs.

Ventilation – the process of bringing air into and out of the lungs (breathing).

Diaphragm – a large sheet of muscle under the rib cage.

Intercostal muscles – the muscles between the ribs.

Thorax – the chest cavity. The area enclosed by the rib cage.

Abdominal cavity – the space within the abdomen that contains the liver, pancreas, stomach and intestines.

Recap Questions

1. Describe the roles of the four chambers of the heart.
2. What are the main components of blood and describe the specific function of each component (red blood cells, white blood cells, platelets, plasma).
3. Explain how red blood cells are adapted for oxygen transport and describe the role of haemoglobin.
4. Describe the pathway of blood through the pulmonary and systemic circulation, starting and ending at the heart.
5. Describe the differences between the structure and function of arteries, veins, and capillaries.
6. Describe the pathway of air from the nose/mouth to the alveoli, naming the key structures involved.
7. Explain how the structure of the alveoli is adapted for efficient gas exchange.
8. What is the process of ventilation, and how does it differ from gas exchange?
9. Describe the mechanism of inhalation, focusing on the role of the diaphragm and intercostal muscles.
10. What is the role of mucus and cilia in the respiratory system, and how do they protect the lungs?

Revision Quiz

1. What is the function of the cell membrane?
2. What is the difference between catabolism and anabolism?
3. What is ATP and why is it important?
4. What is the function of the pituitary gland?
5. Describe the negative feedback mechanism in hormone regulation.
6. What is the function of the lymphatic system?
7. Describe three key risk factors associated with the development of CHD.
8. Name three long-term complications which can result from poorly managed diabetes.
9. What are the primary risk factors for developing breast cancer?

B3 The Nervous system

The central nervous system

The **central nervous system (CNS)** consists of the brain and spinal cord.

The brain is divided into three main parts: the cerebrum, cerebellum, and brainstem:

- The **cerebrum** is the largest part and has many roles like thought, perception, and voluntary movement.
- The **cerebellum** is located at the back of the brain and is primarily responsible for coordinating movement, balance and posture.
- The **brainstem** connects the brain to the spinal cord. It controls vital functions such as breathing, heart rate, and blood pressure.

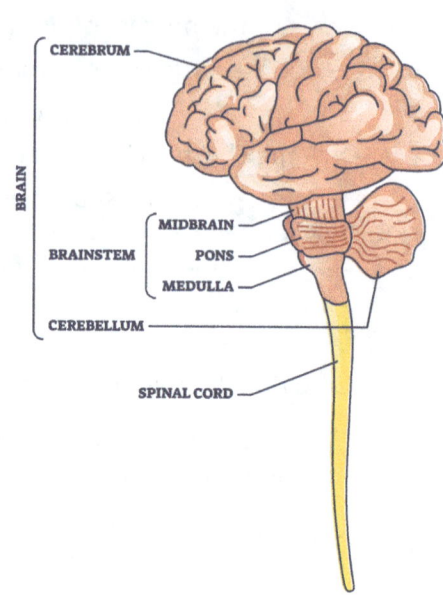

CENTRAL NERVOUS SYSTEM

The **spinal cord** is a long, thin bundle of nerves that extends from the base of the brain to the lower back. It is protected by the **vertebrae** (bones) of the spine.

The spinal cord transmits sensory information from the body to the brain, and motor signals from the brain to the body.

It also plays a role in **reflexes**, which are rapid, involuntary movements that help protect the body from injury.

The peripheral nervous system

The **peripheral nervous system (PNS)** is the network of nerves that connect the central nervous system (brain and spinal cord) to the rest of the body.

It has many functions including:

- **Sensory functions:** Sending information from the senses (sight, hearing, touch, taste, smell) to the brain.
- **Motor functions:** Carrying instructions from the brain to muscles and organs in order to control movement, breathing, digestion, etc.
- **Autonomic functions:** Regulating involuntary processes like heart rate, blood pressure, and body temperature.

Nerves in the PNS connect the CNS to peripheral organs like muscles and glands, transmitting impulses to and from the brain and spinal cord.

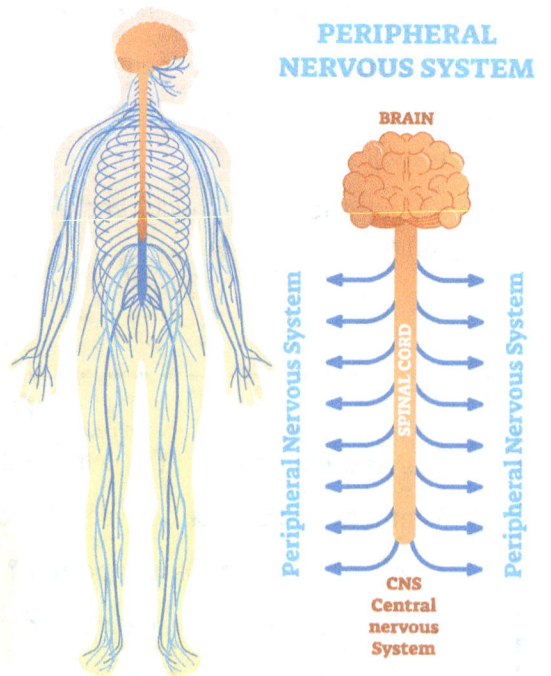

The autonomic nervous system

The **autonomic nervous system** controls involuntary functions such as heart rate, blood pressure, digestion, and body temperature. It is divided into two branches:
- the **parasympathetic nervous system**
- the **sympathetic nervous system**.

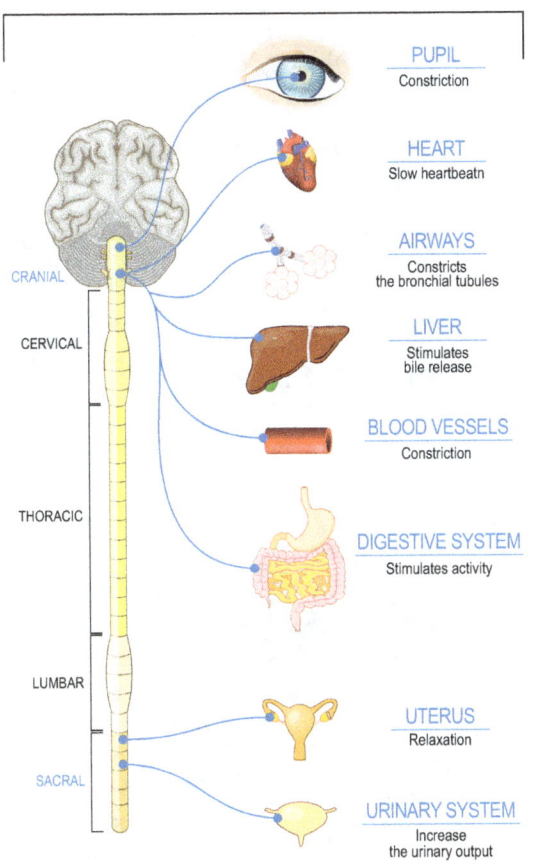
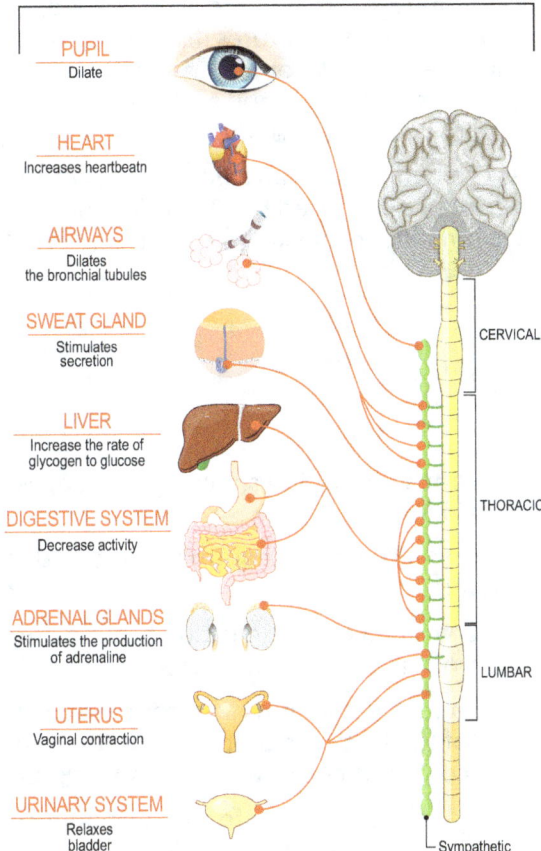

Parasympathetic
- Responsible for the body's 'rest and digest' response.
- Slows heart rate, lowers blood pressure, and stimulates digestion.
- Is activated when the body is at rest and does not need to be alert.

Sympathetic
- Prepares the body for a fight-or-flight response.
- Causes release of adrenaline.
- Increases heart rate, blood pressure, and breathing rate.
- Dilates the pupils and diverts blood flow to the muscles.
- Is activated in response to stress, danger, or excitement.

Perception – the process of interpreting and organising sensory information to understand and make sense of the world around us.

Voluntary movement – any conscious and intentional action by an individual.

Motor signals – messages sent from the brain or spinal cord to muscles, instructing them to contract or relax, thereby producing movement.

Peripheral nervous system (PNS) – the network of nerves that connect the CNS to the rest of the body.

Central nervous system (CNS) – the brain and spinal cord.

Spinal cord – a long, thin bundle of nerves that extends from the base of the brain to the lower back. It is protected by the vertebrae (bones) of the spine.

Autonomic nervous system – controls involuntary functions such as heart rate, blood pressure, digestion, and body temperature.

Parasympathetic nervous system – part of the autonomic nervous system which is in control when the body is at rest (rest and digest).

Sympathetic nervous system – part of the autonomic nervous system which is in control during times of stress or danger (fight or flight).

B4 The endocrine and renal systems

The **endocrine system** is made up of **glands** that secrete **hormones**. The hormones regulate various bodily functions such as metabolism, growth, and reproduction.

The **renal system** is made up of the kidneys and associated structures (like the ureters) and is responsible for filtering waste products from the blood and maintaining fluid balance in the body.

These two systems interact closely, with hormones produced by the endocrine system influencing kidney function.

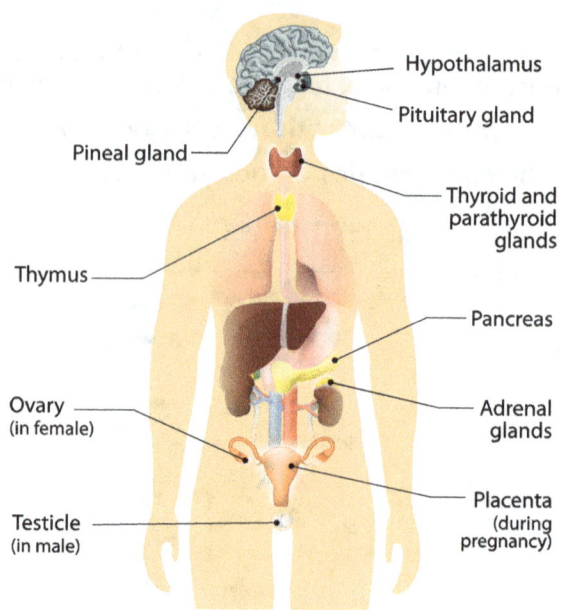

The endocrine system

The hypothalamus

The **hypothalamus** is a small region deep within the brain.

- It plays a key role in controlling the endocrine system.
- It serves as a communication hub, linking the nervous and endocrine systems:
  » It receives information from various parts of the body, including the **brain**, spinal cord, and **peripheral nervous system**.
  » It processes this information and responds by regulating the secretion of hormones from the **pituitary gland**.

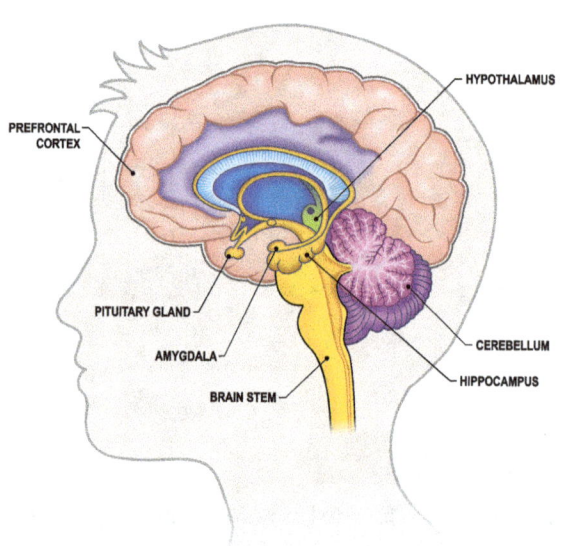

The role of the endocrine system

Control and regulation of growth

The endocrine system releases hormones which regulate growth and development. Several hormones produced by various endocrine glands contribute to this process:

Hormone	Produced by	Effect
thyroid hormone	Thyroid gland	Essential for overall growth and development. Influences metabolic rate, protein synthesis, and bone growth. Insufficient thyroid hormone production can lead to stunted growth and other developmental issues.
testosterone	Testes (males)	Controls male sexual development and growth. Stimulates muscle growth, bone development, and the deepening of the voice. Stimulates the development of **secondary sexual characteristics**, such as facial hair, pubic hair, and increased body mass.

Hormone	Produced by	Effect
Oestrogen and **progesterone**	Ovaries (females)	Responsible for the development of female secondary sexual characteristics, including breast development, widening of the hips, and the onset of menstruation. Progesterone is involved in the preparation of the uterus for pregnancy.
Growth stimulating hormone	Anterior pituitary gland	Stimulates the growth of tissues and organs, including bones and muscles. Particularly important during childhood and adolescence, when rapid growth occurs. Continues to play a role in maintaining bone density and muscle mass throughout life.

Osmoregulation

Osmoregulation is the maintenance of the body's water balance.

- It is controlled by a hormone called **ADH**, which is produced in the hypothalamus.
- The hypothalamus monitors **blood volume** and **solute concentration** (the concentration of dissolvable substances in the blood).

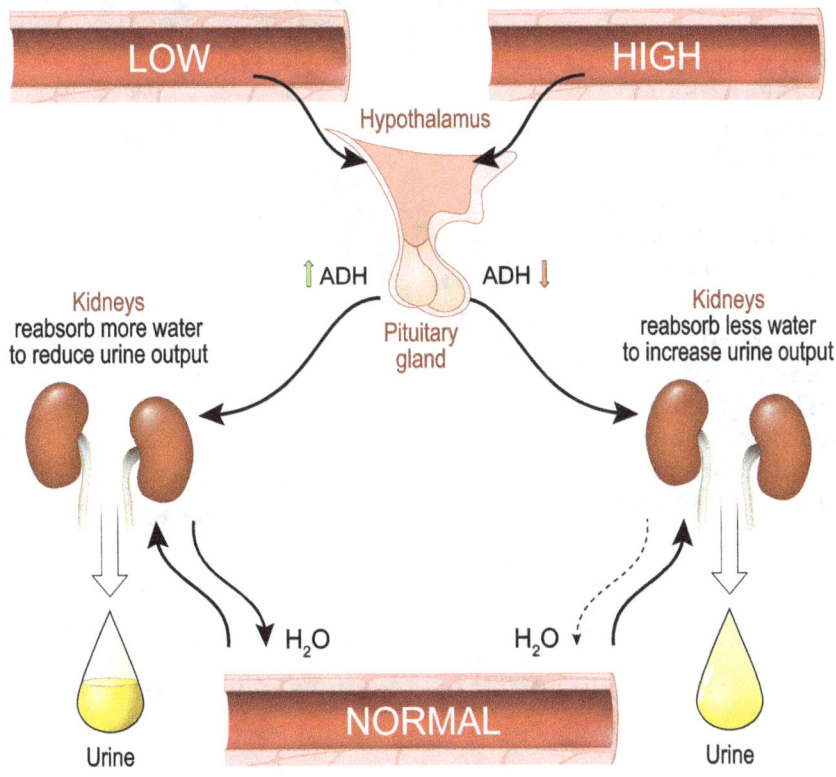

- When **blood volume decreases** or **solute concentration increases** (indicating dehydration), the hypothalamus **releases ADH** into the bloodstream.
- ADH travels to the kidneys, where it acts on the collecting ducts to increase water reabsorption.
- More water is returned to the bloodstream, **reducing urine output** and helping to conserve water.

- When **blood volume increases** or **solute concentration decreases** (indicating excess fluid), the hypothalamus **reduces ADH secretion**.
- **Less water is reabsorbed** by the kidneys
- This allows **more water to be excreted** in the urine.

Regulation of blood sugar

The endocrine system is responsible for maintaining a stable blood glucose level, a process known as **glucoregulation**.

Two hormones, **insulin** and **glucagon**, produced by the **pancreas**, regulate blood glucose levels.

- **Insulin** is secreted by the **beta cells** of the pancreas when **blood glucose levels increase** (e.g. after a meal).
- Insulin acts on target tissues, such as muscle, liver, and adipose (fatty) tissue, causing them to take up glucose and store it.
- In the liver, **insulin converts excess glucose** into **glycogen**, a stored form of glucose.

- **Glucagon** is secreted by the **alpha cells** of the pancreas and has the opposite effect of insulin.
- It is released in response to **low blood glucose levels**, such as during fasting or exercise.
- Glucagon causes the **liver to breakdown glycogen into glucose** and to **synthesise new glucose molecules** from non-carbohydrate sources (amino acids or fatty acids).

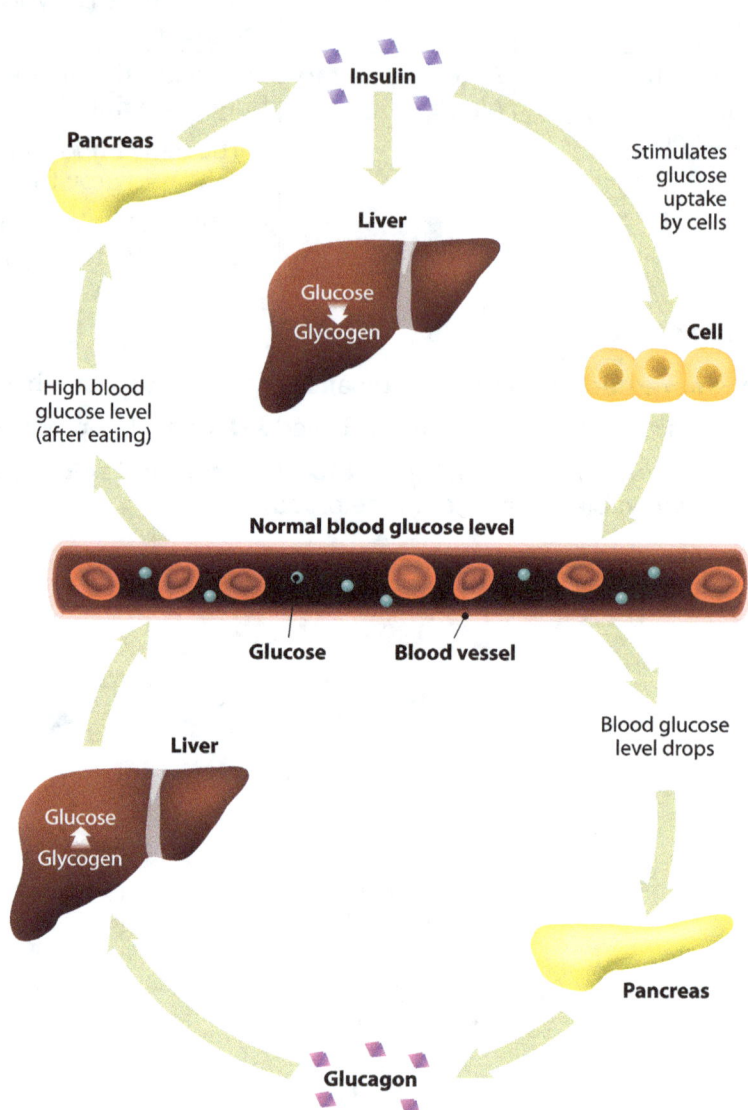

How insulin controls the take-up of glucose by cells

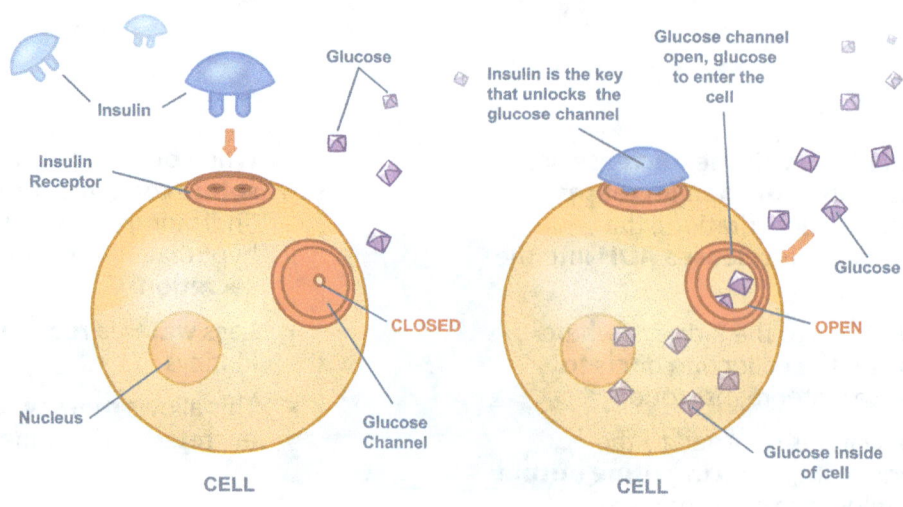

Fight or flight response

The endocrine system is responsible for the body's stress response – often called the **fight or flight** response.

It is designed to enhance the body's ability to respond to danger. When faced with a threat, the hypothalamus sends signals to the adrenal glands causing them to release adrenaline.

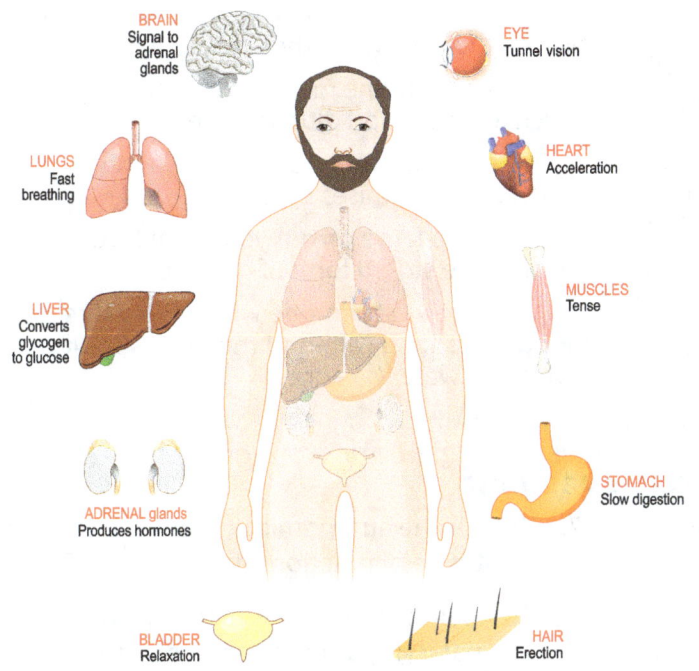

Effects of adrenaline:
- **Increased heart rate and blood pressure**: this makes the heart beat faster and stronger, increasing blood flow to vital organs.
- **Dilated airways**: relaxes the muscles in the airways to increase airflow. This brings more air into the lungs and allows for more oxygen to diffuse into the blood stream.
- **Breakdown of energy stores**: increased breakdown of glycogen in the liver and muscles, releasing glucose into the bloodstream to be used in respiration to release energy.
- **Reduced sensitivity to pain**: this allows individuals to focus on the task at hand.
- Decreased blood flow to digestive system

Regulation of blood pressure

The adrenal glands also play a role in maintaining blood pressure. The **adrenal cortex**, the outer layer of the adrenal gland, produces a hormone called **aldosterone**. Aldosterone regulates blood pressure by altering the body's sodium levels and water balance. By increasing or decreasing the amount of water in the body (and therefore the blood), our bodies can control blood pressure.

Increasing blood pressure:
- When **blood pressure decreases**, specialised cells in the kidneys detect the change and signal the adrenal glands to **increase aldosterone production**.
- Aldosterone acts on the kidneys, mainly in the distal convoluted tubules and collecting ducts, where it causes the reabsorption of sodium ions from the filtrate back into the bloodstream.
- As sodium is reabsorbed, water is also taken up, leading to an increase in blood volume and ultimately, blood pressure.

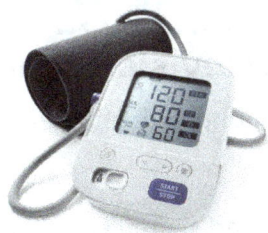

Decreasing blood pressure:
- When **blood pressure increases**, aldosterone secretion is **reduced**.
- This causes more sodium and water to remain in the kidney filtrate, which then forms urine.
- More water and sodium are excreted from the body.
- This leads to a decrease in blood volume and blood pressure.

> **Important terms!**
>
> **Endocrine system** – a system of glands that secrete hormones to control bodily functions.
>
> **Hormones** – chemical messengers which travel through the blood stream to target organs.
>
> **Renal system** – made up of the kidneys and associated structures (like the ureters).
>
> **Hypothalamus** – a small region deep within the brain which plays a key role in coordinating the endocrine system.
>
> **Metabolic rate** – the rate at which the body uses energy to carry out its vital functions, such as breathing, circulating blood, and maintaining body temperature.
>
> **Protein synthesis** - the process by which cells build proteins from individual amino acids, following instructions encoded in DNA.
>
> **Osmoregulation** – the maintenance of the body's water balance.
>
> **ADH** – antidiuretic hormone. The hormone which regulates water levels within the body. It alters the permeability of the collecting ducts in the kidneys.
>
> **Glucoregulation** – the maintenance of a steady blood glucose level in the body.
>
> **Insulin** – a hormone produced in the pancreas which lowers blood glucose levels.
>
> **Glucagon** – a hormone produced in the pancreas which raises blood glucose levels.
>
> **Glycogen** – a large carbohydrate molecule which is the stored form of glucose.
>
> **Aldosterone** – a hormone which regulates blood pressure by altering the body's sodium levels and water balance.

Recap Questions

1. What are the three main components of nervous tissue?
2. Distinguish between the central nervous system (CNS) and the peripheral nervous system (PNS) and explain how they work together.
3. What is the function of sensory neurones, and how do they transmit information from sensory receptors to the CNS?
4. Describe the process by which a sensory stimulus, such as touching a hot pan, triggers a response.
5. What is the function of motor neurones?
6. What are neuroglia (glial cells)? Describe three of their key functions in supporting the nervous system.
7. What is the autonomic nervous system, and what type of functions does it control?
8. Compare the functions of the sympathetic and parasympathetic nervous systems.
9. What are the primary functions of the endocrine system and the renal system, and how do they work together to maintain homeostasis?
10. Describe the role of the hypothalamus in controlling the endocrine system, and how it links the nervous and endocrine systems.
11. What is the function of the thyroid gland, and how does thyroid hormone affect growth and development?
12. Describe the roles of testosterone, oestrogen, and progesterone in growth and development.

Revision Quiz

1. What are the four types of tissue found in the human body?
2. What is homeostasis?
3. What are the common early signs and symptoms of breast cancer?
4. What are the key differences between Alzheimer's disease and vascular dementia?
5. What are the common symptoms of asthma?
6. Describe the key changes that occur in the lungs of a person with emphysema.
7. What are the two main causes of strokes?
8. Explain the role of the liver and gallbladder in digestion.
9. Describe the process of gas exchange in the lungs.

B5 The musculoskeletal system

Ligaments, tendons, cartilage and bone

The musculoskeletal system is made up of **bones**, **muscles**, **tendons**, **ligaments**, and **cartilage** that provides structure, support, and movement to the human body. It acts as a framework, allowing us to stand upright, walk, run, and perform countless other activities.

The musculoskeletal system works with the nervous system to coordinate movement and maintain posture.

Cartilage

- Provides support, structure, and flexibility to the musculoskeletal system.
- Tough yet flexible tissue that can withstand significant forces without breaking.
- Found in various parts of the body, including joints, the nose, the ears, the trachea, and the intervertebral discs (between the vertebrae).
- In joints, cartilage acts as a cushion, reducing friction between bones and preventing wear and tear.

Bone

- Form the rigid framework of the human body, providing structural support, protection for vital organs, and a surface for muscle attachment.
- Composed of a hard, mineralised **matrix** (scaffolding) that gives them strength and rigidity
- Act as anchors for muscles, allowing them to exert force and produce movement.

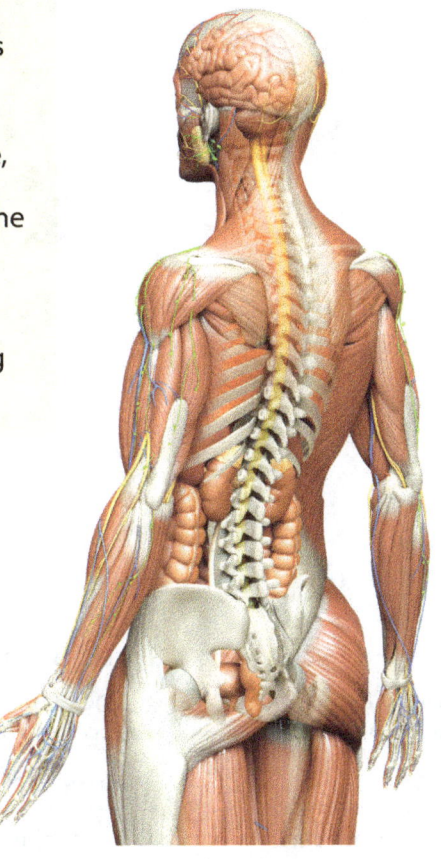

Ligaments

- Tough, fibrous bands of connective tissue
- Connect **bones to bones** to hold the skeleton together.
- Provide stability, support, and structure
- Allow flexibility for a wide range of movements e.g. in the shoulder join they allow a wide range of arm movements.

Tendons

- Connect **muscles to bones**
- Allow muscles to exert force and produce movement.
- Typically composed of dense, fibrous tissue.
- Allow muscles to transmit their force to the skeleton, creating movement.
- Help to stabilise joints and prevent excessive movement that could lead to injury.

Muscle interactions

The human body relies on muscles to produce movement. Muscles often work in groups which allows them to achieve coordinated and controlled motion.

Three main types of muscle interactions are essential for movement:

- **antagonistic pairs**
- **synergistic muscles**
- **fixator muscles**.

Antagonistic pairs

- These are muscles that work in opposition to each other.
- When one muscle contracts, its **antagonist** relaxes, allowing for controlled movement.

For example, the biceps brachii and triceps brachii are antagonistic pairs in the arm.

- Contraction of the biceps brachii flexes the elbow.
- Contraction of the triceps brachii extends the elbow.

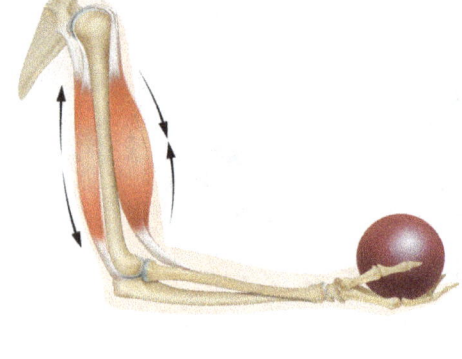
Triceps relaxed. Biceps contracted

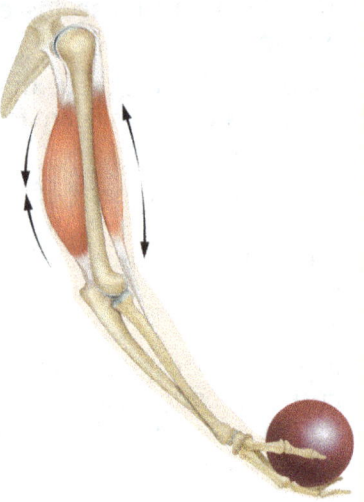
Triceps contracted. Biceps relaxed

Fixator muscles

- These are muscles that stabilise a joint or body part while other muscles produce movement.
  - » For example, when lifting a heavy object, the muscles of the shoulder girdle act as **fixators**, stabilising the shoulder joint and preventing unwanted movement.

Synergistic muscles

- These are muscles that work together to produce a specific movement.
- **Synergists** can assist the primary mover (agonist) in a movement, or they can help to stabilise a joint.
  - » For example, several muscles work together to flex the wrist, including the flexor carpi radialis, flexor carpi ulnaris, and palmaris longus.

Fibrous joints

- Held together by **collagen** fibres.
- Characterised by their **lack of movement** or very limited mobility.
- Provide **stability and support** to the body by firmly connecting bones together.
- Play an essential role in providing structural support and protecting vital organs. For example, the **sutures** of the skull protect the brain.

Cartilaginous joints

- Held together by cartilage.
- Allow for a **limited amount of movement**, making them more flexible than fibrous joints but less mobile than synovial joints.
- Found in areas of the body that require both stability and flexibility, such as the intervertebral discs and the pubic symphysis (the joint which connects the two pubic bones in the pelvis).
- Provides cushioning and allows for a limited amount of movement, such as bending and twisting.

Synovial joints

- The most **movable type of joint** in the human body.
- Characterised by a **fluid-filled joint cavity**, **cartilage**, a **synovial membrane**, and **ligaments**.
- Surrounded by a **fibrous capsule** that provides stability and support.
- Within the joint cavity, cartilage covers the ends of the bones, providing a smooth, low-friction surface for movement.
- Synovial fluid, produced by the synovial membrane, nourishes the cartilage and removes waste products.
- Responsible for a wide range of movements, including flexion, extension, abduction, adduction, rotation, and circumduction.
- Found in most of the major joints in the body, such as the shoulder, elbow, wrist, hip, knee, and ankle.

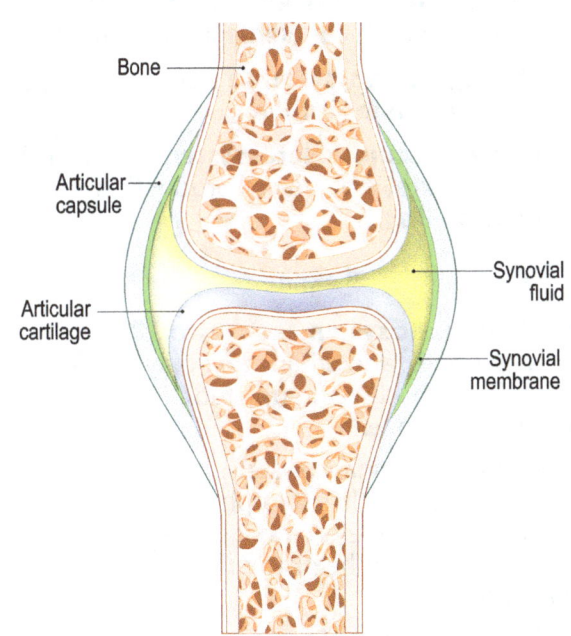

Important terms!

Antagonistic pairs – muscles that work in opposition to each other. When one muscle contracts, its antagonist relaxes, allowing for controlled movement.

Synergistic muscles – muscles that work together to produce a specific movement. They can assist the primary mover, or agonist, in a movement, or they can help to stabilise a joint.

Fixator muscles – muscles that stabilise a joint or body part while other muscles produce movement.

Joint – an area where two or more bones meet.

Fibrous joint – held together by collagen fibres. These joints are fixed and produce little or no movement.

Cartilaginous joints – held together by cartilage. They allow a limited amount of movement.

Synovial joints – the most movable type of joint in the human body. They have a fluid-filled joint cavity, cartilage, a synovial membrane, and ligaments.

B6 The function of further body systems

The immune system

The **immune system** is the body's defence mechanism, responsible for protecting against pathogens (disease causing microorganisms) such as bacteria, viruses, fungi, and parasites.

The body's first line of defence provides a rapid but non-specific response to pathogens. It includes **physical barriers** like the skin and mucous membranes, as well as cells such as neutrophils, macrophages, and natural killer cells.

If the pathogens get past this first line of defence, then a slower but more **specific** response develops over time. It involves the production of antibodies and **T cells**, which can recognise and target specific pathogens.

White blood cells (leukocytes) are a major part of the immune response. There are different types, each with its own specific functions:

- **Neutrophils** are the most common type of white blood cell and are crucial for fighting bacterial infections.
- **Macrophages** are large white blood cells that engulf and destroy pathogens.
- **Natural killer cells** are specialised white blood cells that can kill virus-infected cells and cancer cells.

Antibodies are produced by **B cells**, a type of white blood cell. They bind to antigens, which are foreign molecules on the surface of pathogens. This binding helps to neutralise pathogens and mark them for destruction by other immune cells.

The immune system works alongside other body systems:

- The **lymphatic system** drains fluid from tissues and transports immune cells around the body.
- The **circulatory system** transports immune cells and antibodies throughout the body, allowing them to reach sites of infection or inflammation.
- The **digestive system** is a potential entry point for pathogens and produces **hydrochloric acid** in the stomach to kill them.
- In the **musculoskeletal system** the **bone marrow**, a soft tissue found within bones, is the primary site of blood cell production, including immune cells such as lymphocytes and neutrophils.

The lymphatic system

The **lymphatic system** is a network of vessels, nodes, and organs that play a role in the body's immune function and fluid balance.

It serves as a drainage system, collecting excess fluid (lymph) from tissues and returning it to the bloodstream. This helps to prevent swelling.

- **Lymphatic vessels** are similar to blood vessels and transport **lymphatic fluid** throughout the body.
- **Lymphatic nodes**, located along the lymphatic vessels, act as filters, trapping and destroying pathogens and debris (cellular waste).

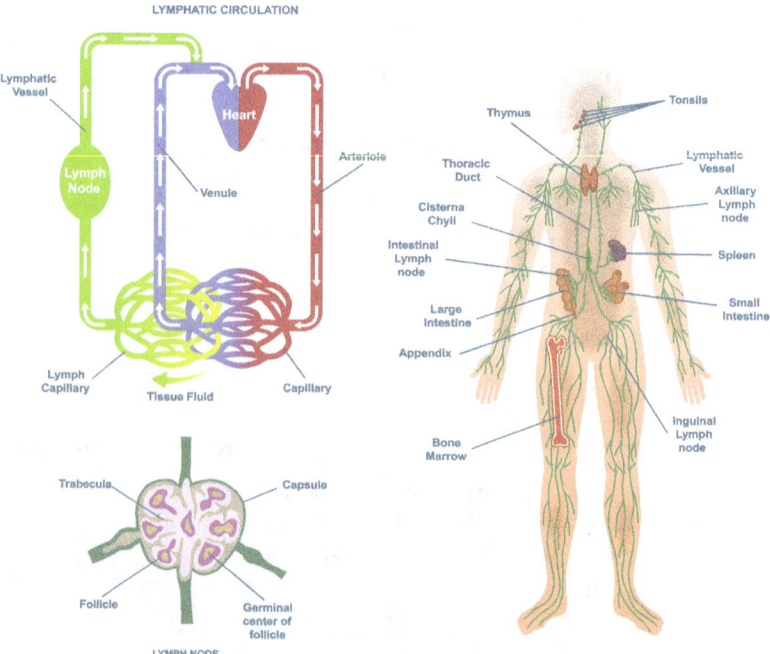

The lymphatic system also plays a crucial role in the immune response by transporting immune cells and antibodies to areas of infection or **inflammation**.

The lymphatic system works with the **digestive system**, as it plays a role in the absorption of fats in the small intestine. Fatty acids and glycerol are first absorbed into lymphatic vessels before being transported to the bloodstream.

The reproductive systems

While the male and female reproductive systems have distinct structures and functions, they share the common goal of producing **gametes** (sperm and eggs) and facilitating fertilisation.

The male reproductive system

- Produces sperm and delivers them to the female reproductive system during sexual intercourse.
- Consists of several key organs, including the **penis** and **testes**.
- The testes are two oval-shaped organs located in the **scrotum**, a sac of skin that hangs outside the body. They produce **sperm** (the male reproductive cells).
- The testes also produce **testosterone**, a hormone that controls male sexual development and function.
- The **penis** is the male organ of sexual intercourse. It contains the urethra, a tube that carries sperm and urine out of the body.
- During sexual arousal, the penis becomes erect, allowing for the delivery of sperm into the vagina.

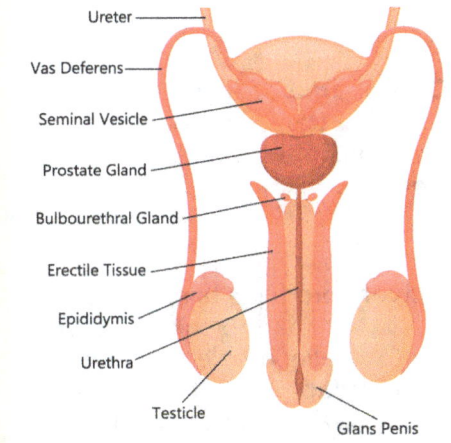

The female reproductive system

- Designed to produce eggs, receive sperm, and grow the developing foetus.
- Consists of several key components, including the **breasts, uterus, ovaries,** and **vagina.**
- The breasts are **mammary glands** that produce milk to nourish a newborn baby. They are made up of glandular tissue and fatty tissue.
- The uterus (womb) is the organ where the developing **foetus** grows. It is lined with a tissue called the **endometrium**, which thickens and prepares for implantation of a **fertilised egg** during the menstrual cycle.
- The ovaries are two small organs located on either side of the uterus. They produce eggs and hormones, including **oestrogen** and **progesterone**, which regulate the menstrual cycle and pregnancy.
- The **vagina** is a muscular tube that connects the uterus to the outside of the body. It serves as the passageway for sperm during sexual intercourse and for the delivery of a baby.

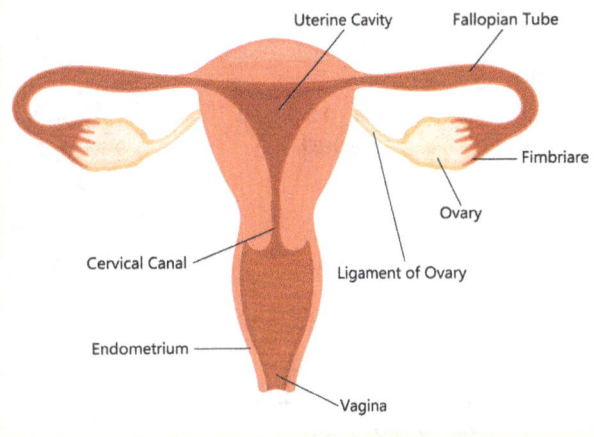

The reproductive systems work alongside other body systems:
- The pituitary gland in the **endocrine system** produces **FSH** and **LH** which control oestrogen secretion and ovulation.
- The **circulatory system** transports hormones throughout the body.
- The **nervous system** controls the physiological processes involved in reproduction, such as sexual arousal and childbirth.
- The **immune system** plays a role in protecting the reproductive organs and preventing infections.

The digestive system

The digestive system breaks food down into small soluble molecules that the body can absorb and use for energy and growth. This process, known as digestion, involves a series of mechanical and chemical processes that occur along the alimentary canal.

Salivary glands - produce saliva, which contains an enzyme (**amylase**) that begins the breakdown of carbohydrates.

Oesophagus - a muscular tube that transports food from the mouth to the stomach.

Stomach - a muscular sac that stores and breaks down food using gastric juices (hydrochloric acid and a protease enzyme called pepsin).

Liver - produces bile, which emulsifies fats (breaks them up into smaller droplets to increase the surface area). The increased surface area then allows **lipase enzyme** to break the fats down faster.

Duodenum - the first part of the small intestine, where most of the digestion and absorption of nutrients occurs.

Gallbladder - stores bile and releases it into the small intestine when needed.

Pancreas - produces digestive enzymes (**lipase**, **proteases** and **carbohydrases**) that aid in the breakdown of fats, proteins, and carbohydrates.

Ileum - the final part of the small intestine, where the remaining nutrients are absorbed.

Anus

Colon (large intestine) - absorbs water and electrolytes before the waste material is eliminated from the body.

The digestive system is closely linked to other body systems:

- **Nervous system:** controls the movement of food through the digestive tract and regulates the secretion of digestive enzymes.
- **Circulatory system:** transports nutrients absorbed from the digestive system to other parts of the body.
- **Endocrine system:** produces hormones that regulate appetite, digestion, and metabolism.
- **Immune system:** plays a role in protecting the digestive tract from pathogens.

> **Study Tips!**
> Make sure you can give a few examples of how the different body systems work with each other. The body systems never work on their own.
>
> Bile isn't an enzyme therefore it doesn't break down fats. Bile **emulsifies** fats (breaks large fat molecules into smaller ones to increase the surface area for lipase to work).
>
> It's easy to get confused between antibodies, antigens and pathogens. Take the time to learn the difference.

Recap Questions

1. What are the main components of the musculoskeletal system, and what are their primary functions?
2. What is cartilage, and where is it found in the body? Explain its function in joints.
3. What are antagonistic muscle pairs, and how do they work together to produce controlled movement? Give an example.
4. Describe the function of synergistic muscles and explain how they contribute to specific movements.
5. What are fixator muscles, and why are they important for coordinated movement and stability? Give an example.
6. How does the musculoskeletal system work in conjunction with the nervous system to achieve movement and maintain posture?
7. Describe the characteristics of fibrous joints and explain their role in providing stability and support.
8. What are the components of a synovial joint, and how does each contribute to its function?
9. Explain the role of synovial fluid and cartilage within a synovial joint.
10. What are the two main components of the immune system, and how do their responses differ?
11. Describe the role of white blood cells (leukocytes) in the immune response and give examples of different types and their specific functions.
12. Explain how antibodies contribute to the adaptive immune response, including their interaction with antigens.
13. How do the lymphatic and circulatory systems work with the immune system to defend the body against pathogens?
14. What role does the musculoskeletal system play in the immune response?
15. What are the main components of the lymphatic system, and what are their functions?
16. Explain how the lymphatic system contributes to fluid balance in the body, and why this is important.
17. Describe the relationship between the lymphatic system and the circulatory system.
18. What is the role of lymph nodes in the immune response?
19. How does the lymphatic system interact with the digestive system?
20. Describe the structure and function of the testes and the penis in the male reproductive system.
21. Explain the roles of the ovaries, uterus, and vagina in the female reproductive system.
22. How do hormones, specifically FSH, LH, oestrogen, and progesterone, regulate the female reproductive system?
23. Describe how the endocrine, circulatory, nervous, and immune systems interact with the reproductive systems.
24. Describe the path food takes through the alimentary canal, naming the key organs and their specific roles in digestion.
25. Explain the functions of the accessory organs (liver, pancreas, gallbladder, salivary glands) and how they contribute to digestion.

> **Important terms!**
> **Pathogen** – a disease-causing organism, such as a bacteria or virus.
> **Antibodies** – a Y-shaped protein created by the immune system to identify and destroy pathogens by binding to antigens.
> **Antigen** – molecules (commonly proteins) that cause an immune response. A pathogen carries antigens on its surface, which triggers an immune response.
> **Emulsify** – The breakdown of large droplets of fat into smaller droplets, which increases their surface area so the fat can be broken down more quickly.
> **Digestion** – The process of breaking larger food molecules into smaller molecules so they can be absorbed into the blood.

Revision Quiz

1. Which organelle is responsible for protein synthesis?
2. What is the 'powerhouse' of the cell, and what process does it carry out?
3. Name three types of connective tissue and give the function of each type.
4. What are the three types of muscle tissue, and where can each be found?
5. What is the difference between arteries and veins?
6. Explain the role of haemoglobin in oxygen transport.
7. What is the function of a neurone?
8. What is the difference between the central nervous system (CNS) and the peripheral nervous system (PNS)?
9. What are the functions of bones?
10. Describe the structure of a synovial joint.
11. What is the role of tendons and ligaments?
12. Describe three primary effects of a stroke on brain function.
13. Name the two main conditions that commonly fall under the umbrella term of COPD.
14. Name two potential complications of COPD.
15. Which type of diabetes is an autoimmune condition?
16. What are the possible long-term effects of poorly controlled asthma?
17. What lifestyle changes can help manage or prevent type 2 diabetes?
18. What are the main causes of dementia?
19. What are the primary ways in which dementia can affect other body systems, including mobility, coordination, and bladder control?
20. What are some of the primary effects of ABI on cognitive function?
21. Describe the main genetic mutations associated with an increased risk of breast cancer.
22. What are the primary effects of bowel cancer on the digestive system?
23. What is the function of the nephron?
24. What are the components of urine?
25. What is the function of the alveoli?
26. What is osmoregulation, and which organ plays a key role in this process?

Assessment practice

1. The diagram shows a cross section of a human heart. Identify structures A, B & C. (3)

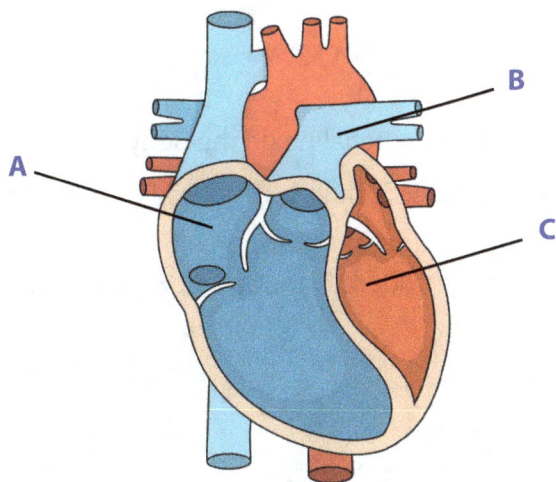

2. Describe the role of valves in maintaining blood flow through the heart. (2)
3. Explain the role of white blood cells in fighting infection. (3)
4. The diagram shows a cross section of the human brain. Identify structures X, Y & Z. (3)

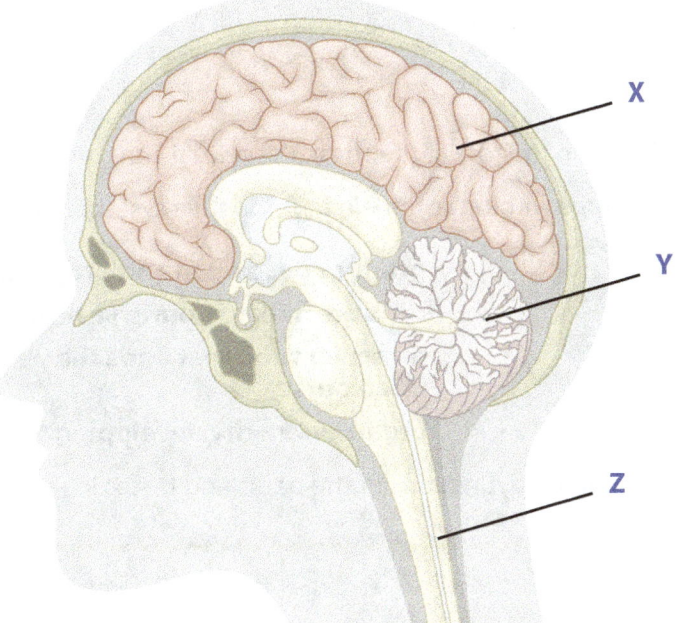

5. Describe the differences between the roles of the sympathetic and parasympathetic nervous system. (4)
6. Circle two hormones associated with control and regulation of growth: (2)

    ADH   testosterone   thyroid hormone   insulin

7. Which cells produce insulin? (1)

    b) alpha

    c) beta

    d) gamma

    e) hypothalamus

8. Describe and explain two effects of adrenaline on the body. (4)

9. Describe what is meant by antagonistic muscles and explain how they bring about movement. (4)

10. The diagram shows a synovial joint. Identify the structures labelled D, E & F. (3)

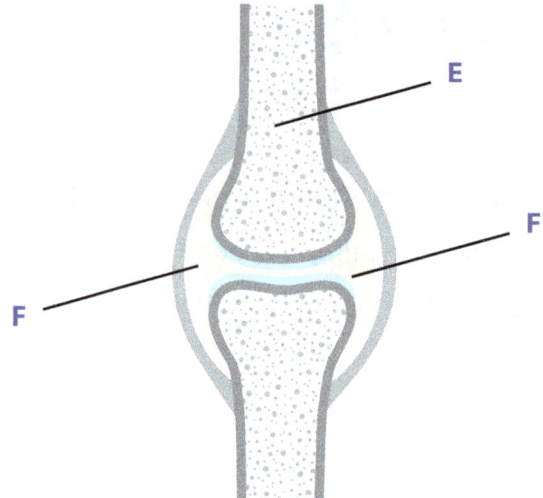

11. Describe and explain the role of the musculoskeletal system in immunity. (5)

12. Link these structures within the female reproductive system to their function. (3)

breasts	produce oestrogen and progesterone
uterus	produce milk to nourish a newborn baby
ovaries	muscular tube that hods the penis during intercourse
vagina	organ where the developing foetus grows

13. Describe and explain the functions of the penis and testes in reproduction. (5)

C Disorders of the body and the effect on body systems

C1 Main disorders of the body systems

Coronary Heart Disease

Coronary heart disease (**CHD**) is a leading cause of death worldwide. It occurs when the **arteries** that supply blood to the heart become **narrowed or blocked** by a buildup of **plaque**. This buildup, known as **atherosclerosis**, can lead to a heart attack or stroke if the blood flow to the heart is significantly reduced or cut off entirely.

Causes of CHD

Atherosclerosis

- Occurs when plaque, a substance composed of cholesterol, fatty substances, cellular waste products, calcium, and fibrin, builds up in the coronary arteries (the arteries that supply blood to the heart).
- This narrows the arteries, reducing blood flow to the heart muscle.
- Over time, the plaque can rupture, leading to blood clots that can block the arteries completely, causing a heart attack.

ATHEROSCLEROSIS STAGES

NORMAL FUNCTIONS
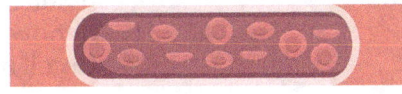

CHOLESTEROL PLAQUE FORMATION
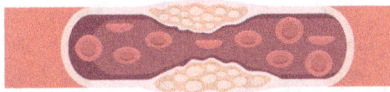

COMPLETE BLOCKAGE
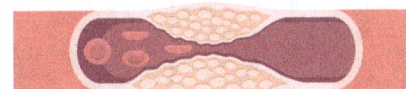

HEART ATTACK
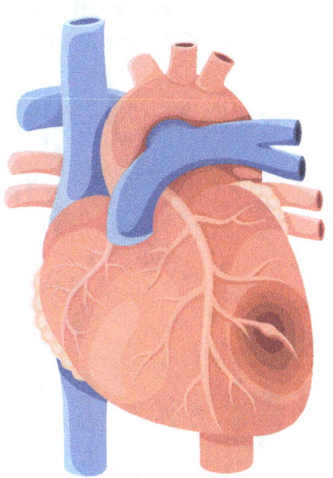

Hypertension (high blood pressure)

- Consistently raised blood pressure puts extra strain on the heart and blood vessels.
- This can lead to damage to the artery walls and lead to the development of atherosclerosis.
- High blood pressure can also increase the risk of blood clots forming in the coronary arteries.

Primary effects of CHD	Secondary effects of CHD
Heart attack: occurs when a coronary artery becomes completely blocked, cutting off blood flow to a portion of the heart muscle. This can cause chest pain, shortness of breath, sweating, nausea, and vomiting. If the blockage is not treated promptly, it can lead to heart muscle damage or death.	**Shortness of breath**: a common symptom of CHD, especially when the heart muscle is weakened or unable to pump blood efficiently. It can be caused by a variety of factors, such as fluid buildup in the lungs or decreased blood flow to the heart.
Angina: occurs when the heart muscle does not receive enough oxygen. It causes chest pain or discomfort. It can happen when the coronary arteries become narrowed, reducing blood flow to the heart. Angina can be a warning sign of a heart attack.	**Dizziness**: can occur if the heart is unable to pump enough blood to the brain. This can lead to a decrease in blood pressure and reduced oxygen supply to the brain.
Heart failure: occurs when the heart muscle is unable to pump enough blood to meet the body's needs. This can be caused by damage to the heart muscle due to a heart attack or other conditions. Heart failure can lead to shortness of breath, fatigue, and swelling in the legs and ankles.	**Nausea and vomiting**: can occur in some individuals with CHD, especially during or after a heart attack. When the heart doesn't work properly, fluid can build up in the liver and stomach, which can cause nausea and loss of appetite.

Stroke

Strokes are a serious neurological condition that occurs when blood flow to the brain is interrupted or reduced. This can lead to damage to brain cells and a range of symptoms, from mild to severe.

Haemorrhagic stroke
- Occurs when a blood vessel in the brain bursts and bleeds.
- Can be caused by a variety of factors, including high blood pressure, **aneurysms**, and blood clotting disorders.
- When a blood vessel ruptures, the blood leaks into the brain tissue which can put pressure on brain tissue and cause damage to brain cells.

Ischaemic stroke
- The most common type of stroke.
- Occurs when a blood vessel that supplies blood to the brain becomes blocked.
- The blockage can be caused by a blood clot (thrombosis) or an embolus (a clot that travels from another part of the body to the brain).
- When a blood vessel is blocked, the brain tissue beyond the blockage becomes deprived of oxygen and nutrients, leading to cell death.

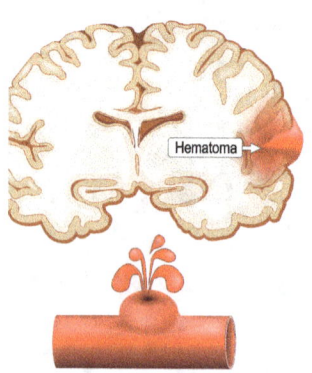

Haemorrhagic stroke — Ruptured aneurysm

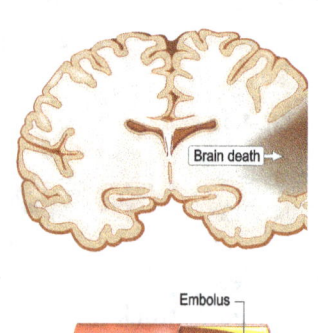

Ischaemic stroke — Thrombosis

Primary effects of a stroke	Secondary effects of a stroke
Brain damage: When blood flow to the brain is interrupted, brain cells can become damaged or die. This damage can lead to neurological problems including weakness or paralysis, difficulty speaking or understanding language, and changes in vision.	**Muscle weakness**: Strokes can cause muscle weakness or paralysis, particularly on one side of the body. This can make it difficult to perform daily activities such as walking, dressing, or eating and can lead to a loss of independence. It can also increase the risk of respiratory infections, such as pneumonia, due to weakened muscles involved in breathing and swallowing.
Bleeding: In haemorrhagic strokes, bleeding into the brain can cause significant damage to brain tissue. The pressure from the blood can compress brain cells and disrupt their function.	**Lack of coordination**: Strokes can also affect coordination, making it difficult to perform tasks that require fine motor skills, such as writing or buttoning clothes.
Clotting: In ischaemic strokes, blood clots can block blood flow to the brain, leading to tissue damage. The clots can also break off and travel to other parts of the brain, causing multiple strokes.	**Dysphasia**: A language disorder that can occur after a stroke. It can affect a person's ability to understand or express language, making communication difficult.

The specific effects of a stroke that a patient will experience will depend on the location of the brain damage:
- a stroke in the left hemisphere of the brain may affect language and speech
- a stroke in the right hemisphere may affect spatial awareness and problem-solving.

Impact on other body systems

- **Cardiovascular system**: The underlying conditions that contribute to strokes, such as high blood pressure and atherosclerosis, can also increase the risk of heart disease. Strokes can also damage the heart muscle, leading to heart failure or **arrhythmias** (irregular heartbeat).
- **Nervous system**: Strokes can disrupt the communication pathways between the brain and other parts of the body, leading to problems with sensation, movement, and coordination. This can affect mood and personality and can impact everything from bladder control to swallowing.

> **Important terms!**
>
> Coronary arteries – the arteries that supply blood to the heart.
>
> Atherosclerosis – a build-up of plaque within the coronary arteries.
>
> Plaque – a substance composed of cholesterol, fatty substances, cellular waste products, calcium, and fibrin.
>
> Hypertension – high blood pressure. A normal blood pressure reading is 120/80 mmHg. Hypertension occurs when the blood pressure is consistently 14/90 mmHg or higher.
>
> Aneurysm – a bulging, weakened area in the wall of a blood vessel, like a balloon.
>
> Thrombosis – a blood clot within a blood vessel.
>
> Embolus – a blood clot which travels from another part of the body to the brain.
>
> Hemisphere – the brain is divided into two halves called hemispheres.
>
> Dysphasia – a language disorder that can occur after a stroke.

Chronic obstructive pulmonary disorder

Chronic obstructive pulmonary disorder (COPD) is a group of lung disorders that make it hard to breathe. COPD happens when the lungs become damaged.

COPD is caused by long term exposure to breathing in harmful substances. The main causes are:

- smoking cigarettes
- breathing in harmful substances, like pollution or chemicals.

Over time, these substances irritate the lungs, causing damage which results in the person developing emphysema and/or chronic bronchitis.

Emphysema

- Develops when cigarette smoke or other harmful substances damage the walls of tiny air sacs in the lungs called alveoli.
- The damage causes the walls of the alveoli to break down, making them bigger and uneven in shape.
- This makes the alveoli less effective, so less oxygen is transferred into the blood, which means cells and organs do not get enough oxygen to work well.

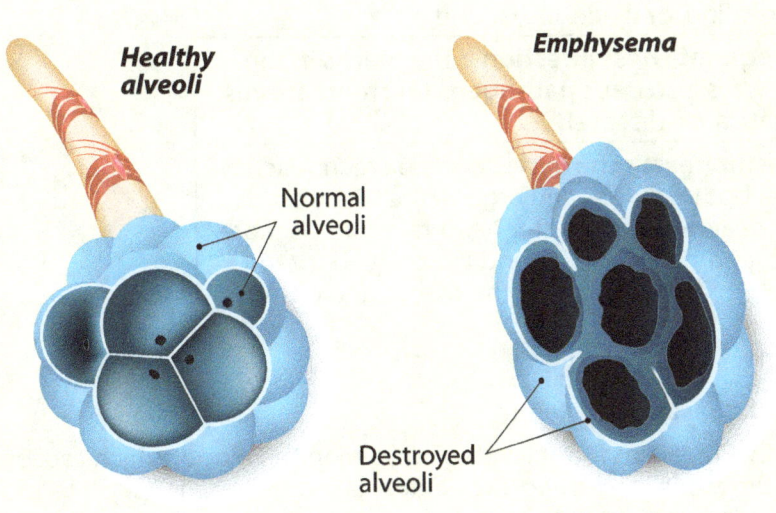

Healthy alveoli — Normal alveoli

Emphysema — Destroyed alveoli

C Disorders of the body and the effect on body systems

Chronic bronchitis

- Develops when your airways (trachea, bronchi, and bronchioles) become permanently inflamed.
- The airways become swollen which make them narrower.
- The airways also start to produce large amounts of mucus.
- This makes it harder to get air in and out of the lungs and leaves the person feeling out of breath.

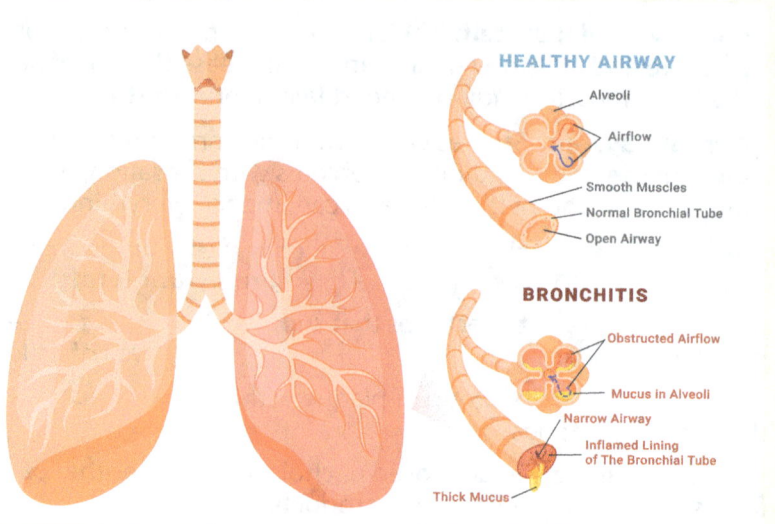

Primary effects of COPD	Secondary effects of COPD
Persistent cough: Coughing is the way in which our airways try to clear out mucus. People with COPD cough a lot because their airways continually make too much mucus.	**Weight loss:** Breathing with COPD uses a lot of energy, so your body burns more calories just to breathe. COPD can also make you feel less hungry because of inflammation in your body. Over time, if the calories you are eating are less than the calories you are burning, you can start to lose weight.
Being out of breath: The mucus clogs the airways making it harder for air to move in or out. Inflammation in the airways also makes them narrower which makes it much harder to move air in and out of the lungs.	**Muscle weakness:** As COPD makes it hard to breathe people with COPD often become physically inactive, as they will tire easily when doing physical activities. This often means that they will stop doing simple daily activities like walking. Over time, this makes their muscles weaker.
Wheezing: Happens when the airways are inflamed or blocked with mucus. The air that is being inhaled (or exhaled) is being forced through a narrower space. This creates the whistling, or wheezing, sound.	**Loss of mobility**: This is due to a combination of factors. Shortness of breath, weight loss and muscle weakness all make a person less likely to be mobile.
Frequent chest infections: The mucus in the airways also traps **pathogens** (microorganisms that cause disease).	
Faster heart rate: Because less oxygen reaches the body's tissues and organs, the heart needs to beat faster. The faster heart rate pumps more oxygen-rich blood around the body to try to deliver more oxygen to the tissues and organs.	

Impact on other body systems

Cardiovascular system:

- COPD causes lower levels of oxygen in the blood, which causes the heart rate to increase. Over time, this can lead to a condition called pulmonary hypertension (high blood pressure in the pulmonary arteries).
- The long-term inflammation caused by COPD can also cause the development of atherosclerosis, a condition where plaque builds up inside the arteries, restricting blood flow to the heart and to the brain. This increases the risk of cardiovascular disease like coronary artery disease, heart attack and strokes.

Digestive system:
- The main impact of COPD on the digestive system is weight loss and malnutrition.
- The chronic coughing due to COPD can also weaken the muscles that control the opening between the oesophagus and the stomach. This can lead to a condition known as gastroesophageal reflux disease (GERD), where stomach acid can move into the oesophagus causing heartburn and damage to the oesophagus.

Musculoskeletal system:

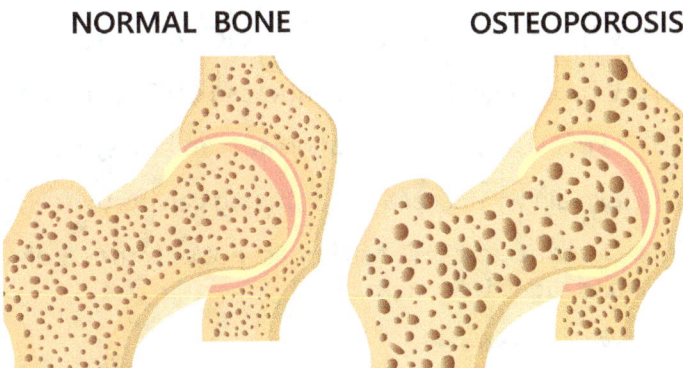

- The reduced lung function in COPD results in reduced physical activity, muscle weakness and eventually **muscular atrophy** (muscle wasting). This will lead to even less physical activity and reduced mobility.
- Reduced physical activity, poor nutrition and the use of steroid medication can lead to a decrease in bone density. This puts the individual at greater risk of developing osteoporosis and bone fractures.

Study Tips!
- 'Chronic' means a condition which is long term.
- All of our organ systems work together to maintain proper functioning of the body. Make sure you can describe not only the impact has on the specific body system but also the impact each of the disorders has on other body systems.

Important terms!

Chronic – a long-term disorder which gets worse over time.

Obstructive – restricting the movement of air in and out of the lungs.

Pulmonary – anything relating to or affecting the lungs.

Chronic obstructive pulmonary disorder (COPD) – a group of lung disorders that make it hard to breathe.

Emphysema – a type of COPD characterised by damage to the alveoli.

Alveoli – the small air sacs in the lungs where gas exchange occurs.

Chronic bronchitis – a type of COPD with long-term inflammation of the airways in the lungs, resulting in a productive cough (coughing up mucus).

Pulmonary hypertension – where the blood pressure in the pulmonary artery (the artery which carries blood from the heart to the lungs) becomes dangerously high. The extra strain on the heart can also cause the right ventricle to weaken, leading to heart failure.

Gastroesophageal reflux disease (GERD) – the muscles that control the opening between the oesophagus and the stomach weaken, leading to stomach acid moving into the oesophagus, causing heartburn and damage to the oesophagus.

Recap Questions

1. What is coronary heart disease (CHD), and what is the underlying process that usually causes it?
2. Describe the process of atherosclerosis and explain how it can lead to a reduction or blockage of blood flow in the coronary arteries.
3. Explain how hypertension increases the risk of developing CHD.
4. What is a heart attack, and how is it related to CHD?
5. What is heart failure, and how can CHD contribute to its development?
6. Explain why shortness of breath can be a symptom of CHD.
7. Explain why nausea and vomiting can occur as a consequence of CHD.
8. Describe how CHD can impact not only the cardiovascular system but also the respiratory and digestive systems.
9. What is a stroke?
10. Describe the two main types of stroke, ischaemic and haemorrhagic, and explain the underlying mechanism of each.
11. What are the primary effects of a stroke on the brain, regardless of the type?
12. How can the location of brain damage from a stroke influence the specific primary effects a patient might experience? Give an example.
13. List four potential secondary effects of a stroke that can impact a person's daily life.
14. Explain why muscle weakness and a lack of coordination are common secondary effects following a stroke.
15. What is dysphasia, and how can it affect individuals who have had a stroke?
16. Why can strokes increase the risk of respiratory infections like pneumonia?
17. What does the acronym COPD stand for, and what are the three key characteristics that define this group of lung disorders?

Revision Quiz

1. What is the difference between simple and compound epithelial tissue?
2. What are the reactants and products of aerobic respiration?
3. What is the purpose of the coronary arteries?
4. Explain the role of insulin and glucagon in blood glucose regulation.
5. What are the functions of T cells and B cells in the immune system?
6. What are the functions of the large intestine?
7. What is the main difference between type 1 and type 2 diabetes in terms of insulin production?
8. What are the early symptoms of Alzheimer's disease?
9. What are the effects of bowel cancer on the cardiovascular system?
10. What are the two main categories of ABI, and what are the key differences between them?
11. How might ABI affect sensory functions, such as vision or hearing?

Asthma

Asthma is a chronic lung condition that is characterised by inflammation and narrowing of the airways, leading to wheezing, coughing, shortness of breath, and chest tightness.

Asthma is caused by a combination of genetic and environmental factors. Common triggers include:

- **allergens** such as pollen, dust mites, and mould
- **irritants** such as cigarette smoke, air pollution, and strong odours (e.g. perfumes)
- respiratory infections
- exercise.

These triggers can cause inflammation and muscle spasms in the airways, leading to the symptoms of asthma.

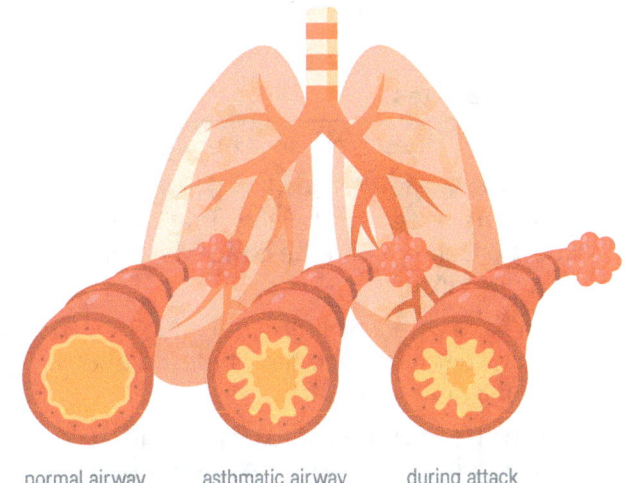

normal airway   asthmatic airway   during attack

Primary effects of asthma	Secondary effects of asthma
Shortness of breath: This is a common symptom of asthma, and it occurs when the airways become narrowed, making it difficult to breathe.	**Anxiety and depression**: Chronic asthma can lead to anxiety and depression, as individuals may worry about having an asthma attack or feel limited by their condition.
Wheezing: Wheezing is a high-pitched whistling sound that occurs when air is forced through the narrowed airways.	**Pneumonia**: People with asthma are at a higher risk of developing pneumonia, a lung infection.
Tight chest: As the airways constrict the chest feels tight.	**Developmental delays in children**: Poor sleep and reduced physical activity can cause delays in growth and development.
Coughing: This happens to try to remove the extra mucus in the airways.	
During an asthma attack the person will feel breathless, will have a faster heart rate and breathing rate, and may feel dizzy, drowsy and confused. Due to lack of oxygen, they may faint. Blue lips and fingers are a sign of severe oxygen deprivation and require urgent medical attention.	

Impact on other body systems

- **Respiratory system**: As well as an increased risk of infection, people with asthma may get respiratory failure. This is where the airways become so narrowed that the lungs can't deliver enough oxygen to the body.
    - » Asthma can also contribute to **sleep apnoea**, a condition where breathing is interrupted during sleep, causing the person to wake up several times a night. This can lead to fatigue and daytime sleepiness.
- **Cardiovascular system**: When the lungs are struggling to get enough oxygen, the heart must work harder to pump blood. This can put strain on the heart and lead to conditions such as high blood pressure, heart rate irregularities, and heart failure.
    - » The chronic inflammation associated with asthma can also contribute to the development of atherosclerosis, a condition where plaque builds up in the arteries, increasing the risk of heart attack and stroke.

Diabetes – type 1 and type 2

Diabetes is a chronic condition that occurs when the body cannot produce enough **insulin** or cannot effectively use the insulin it produces.

Insulin is the hormone that helps to regulate blood sugar levels. When blood sugar levels are too high, it can damage the body's organs and tissues. There are two main types of diabetes: **Type 1 diabetes** and **Type 2 diabetes**.

Type 1 diabetes	Type 2 diabetes
• The body doesn't produce enough insulin. • An **autoimmune disorder** – the body's immune system mistakenly attacks and destroys the cells in the pancreas which produce insulin. • Can have a genetic link – individuals with family members who have type 1 diabetes are at a higher risk. • Exposure to viruses or toxins may also trigger the autoimmune response in susceptible individuals.	• Occurs when the body either doesn't produce enough insulin or doesn't use insulin effectively. • Primarily caused by lifestyle factors. • Risk factors include obesity, a sedentary lifestyle, and a diet high in unhealthy foods. • Results in **insulin resistance** - a condition where the body's cells become less responsive to insulin. • Over time, the pancreas can lose its ability to produce enough insulin to meet the body's needs, resulting in high blood sugar levels.

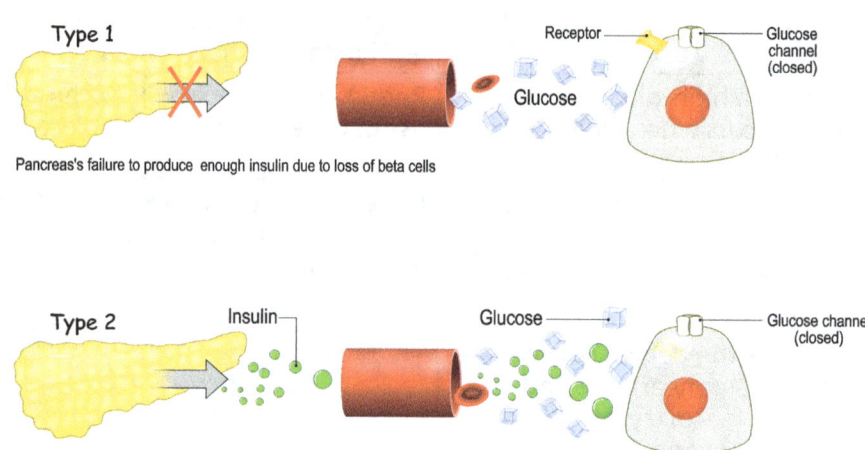

Pancreas's failure to produce enough insulin due to loss of beta cells

Insulin resistance contributes to high glucose levels in the blood

Primary effects of diabetes	Secondary effects of diabetes
Weight change: Uncontrolled blood sugar levels can cause fluctuations in weight. For example, **hypoglycaemia** (low blood sugar) can cause sweating and shaking which can cause weight loss.	**Heart disease and stroke**: High blood sugar levels can damage the blood vessels, leading to atherosclerosis, a condition where plaque builds up in the arteries. This can increase the risk of heart attack and stroke.
Eye problems: High blood sugar levels can cause the lens in the eye to become cloudy leading to cataracts. It can also cause damage to the nerves in the retina leading to diabetic retinopathy which can result in blindness.	**Nerve damage (neuropathy)**: High blood sugar levels can damage the nerves throughout the body, leading to numbness, tingling, pain, and weakness.
Increased thirst: The body may try to eliminate excess glucose through the urine, which can lead to dehydration and increased thirst.	**Foot problems**: Nerve damage and poor blood flow to the feet can increase the risk of developing foot ulcers and infections. These infections can be difficult to treat and can sometimes lead to amputation.

Primary effects of diabetes	Secondary effects of diabetes
Increased hunger: High blood sugar levels can also affect the body's ability to use glucose for energy, leading to increased hunger.	**Miscarriage and stillbirth**: Women with diabetes are at a higher risk of experiencing miscarriage or stillbirth. Diabetes can increase the risk of giving birth to a baby with birth defects.
Mood changes: Fluctuating blood sugar levels can cause mood changes, such as irritability, depression, and anxiety.	**Kidney problems**: High blood sugar levels can damage the kidneys. This is known as diabetic nephropathy. Over time, diabetic nephropathy can lead to kidney failure, which may require dialysis or a kidney transplant.
Tiredness: When blood sugar levels are high, the body's cells may not be able to use glucose for energy efficiently, leading to fatigue.	**Sexual problems**: Nerve damage can lead to erectile dysfunction in men and decreased sexual desire or arousal in women. In women, diabetes can cause vaginal dryness and infections. High blood sugar levels can affect hormone production, which can also contribute to sexual problems.
Itching: Due to dry skin caused by dehydration.	
Thrush infections: High sugar levels can lead to an overgrowth of yeast-like fungi in the mouth, vagina, or skin folds.	
Slow-healing cuts and wounds: High blood sugar levels can impair blood flow and wound healing, making it difficult for cuts and wounds to heal properly.	

Impact on other body systems

Cardiovascular system:
- Diabetes can damage blood vessels, increasing the risk of heart disease and stroke.
- High blood sugar levels can contribute to atherosclerosis, a condition where plaque builds up in the arteries, narrowing them and reducing blood flow. This can increase the risk of heart attack and stroke.

Nervous system:
- High blood sugar levels can damage the nerves throughout the body, leading to numbness, tingling, pain, and weakness.
- Neuropathy can affect the nerves in the feet, hands, legs, and other parts of the body. In severe cases, neuropathy can lead to foot ulcers and infections, which may require amputation.

Immune system:
- Diabetes can weaken the immune system, making individuals more susceptible to infections.
- High blood sugar levels can impair the function of white blood cells, which are essential for fighting infections.
- Diabetes can also damage blood capillaries, making it difficult for immune cells to reach the site of infections.

Digestive system:
- High blood sugar levels can slow down the digestive process, leading to constipation.

> Diabetes – a chronic condition that occurs when the body cannot produce enough insulin or cannot effectively use the insulin it produces.
>
> Insulin – the hormone that helps to regulate blood sugar levels.
>
> Type 1 diabetes – an autoimmune disorder where the body doesn't produce any insulin.
>
> Type 2 diabetes – occurs when the body either doesn't produce enough insulin or doesn't use insulin effectively. Primarily caused by lifestyle factors.
>
> Insulin resistance – a condition where the body's cells become less responsive to insulin.
>
> Neuropathy – nerve damage to the peripheral nervous system (nerves outside the brain and spinal cord).

- Diabetes can damage the nerves in the digestive system, causing **gastroparesis**, a condition where the stomach empties slowly. This can lead to nausea, vomiting, and bloating.

Reproductive system:
- In men, diabetes can lead to erectile dysfunction.
- In women, diabetes can cause vaginal dryness and infections. Diabetes can also increase the risk of complications during pregnancy, such as miscarriage and stillbirth.

Dementia – Alzheimer's disease and vascular dementia

Dementia is a progressive brain disorder that causes a decline in cognitive function. It can affect memory, thinking, language, and behaviour. There are many types of dementia, but two of the most common are **Alzheimer's disease** and **vascular dementia**.

Alzheimer's disease
- Characterised by a buildup of abnormal protein deposits within and around brain cells.
- These deposits, known as **amyloid plaques**, disrupt the normal functioning of brain cells and lead to their death.

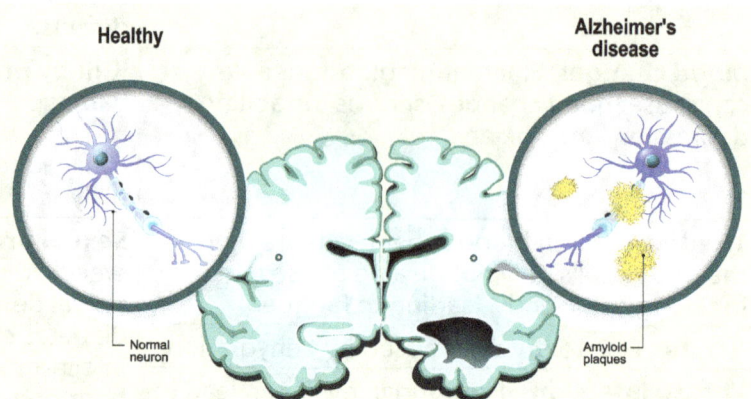

Vascular dementia
- Caused by reduced blood flow to the brain, often due to narrowing of blood vessels, strokes, or **transient ischaemic attacks** (TIAs)
- The arteries that supply blood to the brain can become narrowed due to atherosclerosis. This narrowing can restrict blood flow and oxygen supply to brain cells, leading to damage and cognitive decline.
- Strokes occur when a blood vessel in the brain becomes blocked or bursts, cutting off blood flow to a specific area of the brain. This can cause significant brain damage and lead to cognitive decline.
- TIAs are mini-strokes that last for a short period of time. Multiple TIAs can lead to cumulative brain damage and contribute to vascular dementia.

Primary effects of dementia	Secondary effects of dementia
Memory loss: often the first symptom of dementia and can involve difficulty remembering recent events, names, or faces. As the condition progresses, individuals may also have trouble remembering long-term memories.	**Slowness of thought and confusion**: individuals may experience a decline in their thinking speed and ability to process information. They may become easily confused or have difficulty following conversations.
Difficulty with problem-solving: People with dementia may struggle to solve problems or complete tasks that they used to find easy. This can include difficulties with planning, organising, and sequencing tasks.	**Severe personality changes**: Dementia can lead to significant changes in personality and behaviour. Individuals may become withdrawn, irritable, or anxious. They may also exhibit inappropriate or impulsive behaviour.
Language difficulties: Dementia can affect language skills, making it difficult to find the right words, understand conversations, or follow complex instructions.	**Problems concentrating**: People with dementia often struggle to concentrate and focus on tasks. They may find it difficult to follow conversations or complete simple activities.
Changes in mood and behaviour: As dementia progresses, individuals may experience changes in mood and behaviour, including irritability, anxiety, depression, or agitation.	**Difficulties swallowing or coughing**: Dementia can affect the muscles involved in swallowing and coughing, increasing the risk of choking or aspiration. This can lead to malnutrition and other health problems, such as aspiration pneumonia.

Primary effects of dementia	Secondary effects of dementia
Disorientation: Individuals with dementia may become confused or disoriented, particularly in unfamiliar surroundings.	**Depression**: The cognitive decline and emotional challenges associated with dementia can lead to feelings of sadness, hopelessness, and isolation.
	Incontinence: Dementia can affect the body's ability to control bladder and bowel functions, leading to incontinence.

Impact on other body systems

Nervous system:

- People with dementia may experience motor problems, such as difficulty walking, balance problems, or tremors.
- They may also have difficulty controlling their bladder or bowels.

Cardiovascular system:

- Individuals with dementia are at increased risk of heart disease and stroke, which can be caused by factors such as high blood pressure, high cholesterol, and diabetes. These conditions can further damage the brain and accelerate cognitive decline.

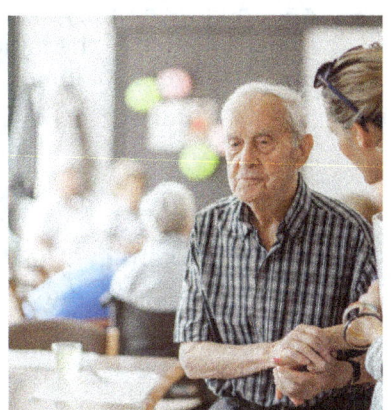

Respiratory system:

- Individuals with dementia may have difficulty swallowing or coughing, which can increase the risk of choking or aspiration. This can lead to respiratory infections and other complications.
- Dementia can affect the muscles involved in breathing, making it more difficult to take deep breaths.

Important terms!

Dementia – a progressive brain disorder that causes a decline in cognitive function. It can affect memory, thinking, language, and behaviour.

Alzheimer's disease – a type of dementia which is characterised by a buildup of abnormal protein deposits (called amyloid plaques) within and around brain cells.

Vascular dementia – caused by reduced blood flow to the brain, often due to narrowing of blood vessels, strokes, or transient ischaemic attacks (TIAs).

Transient ischaemic attacks (TIAs) – mini-strokes that last for a short period of time. Multiple TIAs can lead to cumulative brain damage and contribute to vascular dementia.

Aspiration – the accidental entry of food, liquid, or other foreign material into the lungs or airways.

Acquired brain injury – traumatic and non-traumatic

Acquired brain injuries (**ABI**) happen when the brain is damaged after birth. There are two main causes of acquired brain injury: traumatic and non-traumatic.

Traumatic brain injury

- Occurs when the head is hit hard, like in a road traffic accident, during an assault, or as a result of a fall.
- The effects of a traumatic injury on the brain vary depending on the type of injury, location of the injury, and the severity of injury.

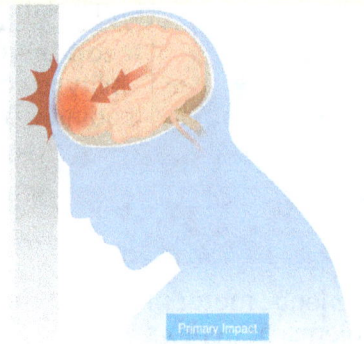
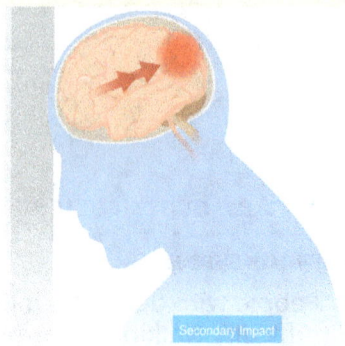

Non-traumatic brain injury

- Does not involve a physical blow to the head.
- Non-traumatic brain injuries can occur due to:
  » having a stroke
  » infections like meningitis
  » lack of oxygen (for example during drowning or suffocation)
  » disease e.g. tumours.

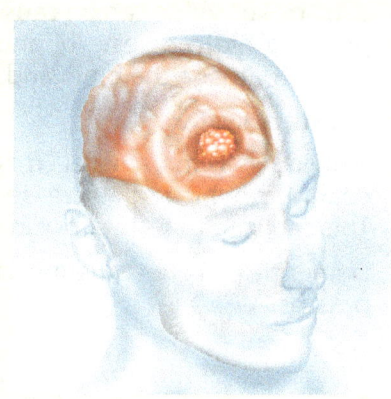

Primary effects of brain injury	Secondary effects of brain injury
Primary effects occur immediately after the injury has happened and will vary depending on the severity and location of the injury	Secondary effects develop over the days and weeks following the initial injury and will vary depending on the severity and location of the injury.
Concussion: A concussion is a result of mild traumatic brain injury. Concussions are often due to a blow to the head, a sudden impact, or violent shaking of the head and upper body. A concussion causes the brain to experience a temporary disruption in its normal functioning.	**Headaches and dizziness**: Inflammation and swelling in the brain can cause the person to suffer from headaches. Bleeding in the brain can result in increased pressure (increased intracranial pressure) which can press on nerves, brain tissue and blood vessels, causing headache pain and feelings of dizziness.
Unconsciousness: This is where a person is not aware of their surroundings and does not respond to an external stimulus such as sound or lights.	**Memory loss**: Memory loss is a common secondary effect. Damage to the frontal lobes and hippocampus could mean that the individual might have problems remembering past events or creating new memories.
Amnesia: Amnesia is a partial or complete loss of memory. It can affect short-term memory, long-term memory, or both. Amnesia may be temporary or permanent.	**Fatigue**: Can result from a combination of physical, cognitive, and emotional factors. Injury to the brain can result in normal processes like the sleep cycle and metabolism being disrupted. The brain uses a lot of energy coping with these effects of the injury

Primary effects of brain injury	Secondary effects of brain injury
Damage to blood vessels in the brain: Both physical trauma and non-traumatic injury can lead to bleeding within the brain. The force of physical trauma can cause blood vessels to rupture or tear. A stroke can be caused when a blood vessel ruptures in the brain.	**Physical and developmental delays in children**: The full effects of the injury are often not seen until the individual starts to use particular skills. Some fine motor skills, for example writing and drawing, develop between the ages of 3-6 years.
Coma: A coma is a deep state of unconsciousness where a person is completely unresponsive and cannot be wakened. 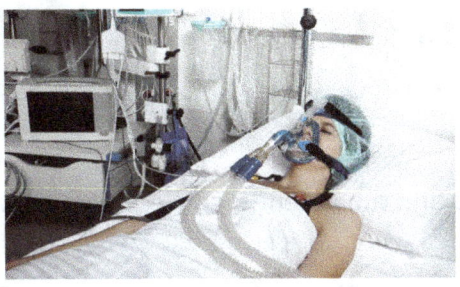	**Cognitive impairments**: Cognitive processes include thinking, reasoning, and making judgements. Someone with a brain injury may process information more slowly or find it difficult to stay focused on a task.
	Sensory impairments: Acquired brain injuries can lead to various sensory impairments, including changes in vision, hearing, taste, smell, and touch.
	Physical impairments: Acquired brain injuries can result in nerve damage, muscle weakness, coordination difficulties and paralysis.
	Irritability: Damage to the frontal lobes or limbic system can result in the individual being unable to process emotions correctly. Cognitive impairments may lead to frustration and anger at not being able to perform simple tasks.
	Sleep disturbance: Injury to the brain can result in normal processes like the sleep-wake cycle being disrupted. This could lead to the individual struggling to fall asleep, stay asleep or achieve deep sleep
	Personality changes: The brain regulates emotions, controls behaviours and social interactions. Damage to the frontal lobe can lead to impulsive behaviour, poor judgement, and irritability. Damage to the limbic system in the brain can result in emotional instability, mood swings and difficulty regulating emotions

Impact on other body systems

Nervous system:
- Damage to the brain may result in some of the sensory impulses from the peripheral nervous system not getting through to the brain, or prevent motor impulses from being sent to the muscles or glands.

Cardiovascular system:
- Brain injury can cause imbalances in heart rate and blood pressure. People who sustain a brain injury have an increased risk of developing chronic cardiovascular disease.

Respiratory system:
- Damage to the brainstem (which controls breathing) could lead to changes in breathing depth or could result in an irregular breathing pattern.
- A brain injury can cause paralysis in the breathing muscles (diaphragm and intercostal muscles), preventing the lungs from inflating.

> **Important terms!**
> Neuromuscular junctions – the site where a motor neurone transmits a nerve impulse to a muscle fibre.
> Motor areas – regions of the cerebral cortex responsible for planning, controlling, and carrying out voluntary movements.

Musculoskeletal system:
- Nerve endings are found in every muscle in our bodies at the neuromuscular junctions. Damage to the motor areas in the brain can lead to muscle weakness or paralysis, making it difficult to control movements.

Recap Questions

1. What are the four main symptoms of asthma?
2. Describe the interaction between genetic and environmental factors in the development of asthma.
3. List four common environmental triggers that can induce asthma symptoms.
4. What are the primary effects of asthma on breathing?
5. During a severe asthma attack, what are some of the serious and potentially life-threatening symptoms that can occur?
6. Describe three potential secondary effects of living with chronic asthma.
7. Explain why individuals with asthma have a higher risk of developing pneumonia.
8. Describe how can asthma lead to respiratory failure.
9. Describe how asthma can contribute to sleep apnoea and the potential consequences of this condition.
10. Explain how asthma can also impact the cardiovascular system.
11. Describe the differences in the causes of Type 1 and Type 2 diabetes.
12. What are the lifestyle risk factors associated with the development of Type 2 diabetes? What is insulin resistance?
13. Describe three common symptoms of diabetes related to changes in blood sugar levels and their effects on the body.
14. Explain how high blood sugar levels can lead to vision problems such as blurred vision, cataracts, and diabetic retinopathy.
15. List five serious secondary effects or long-term complications that can arise from uncontrolled diabetes.
16. How does diabetes increase the risk of heart disease and stroke?
17. Explain how high blood sugar levels can lead to nerve damage (neuropathy) and potential consequences such as foot problems.
18. Describe how diabetes can impact at least three other body systems.

Revision Quiz

1. What are the three types of muscle tissue, and where can each be found?
2. What factors influence Basal Metabolic Rate (BMR)?
3. Explain the role of the diaphragm in breathing.
4. Explain the role of insulin and glucagon in blood glucose regulation.
5. Explain the concept of immunological memory.
6. Where is testosterone produced?
7. What lifestyle changes can a person make to reduce their risk of developing CHD?
8. How effect does exercise have om asthma? How can people with asthma manage it?
9. What are the common early symptoms of bowel cancer?
10. What are the primary effects of bowel cancer on the digestive system?

Breast Cancer

Breast cancer is uncontrolled growth of abnormal cells in the breast tissue. A combination of genetic, lifestyle, and environmental factors all play a role in the development of this disease.

1. **Genetic factors**: Some women may have a genetic predisposition to breast cancer. This means that they inherit genes that increase their risk of developing the disease. These genes (BRCA genes) are known as cancer-risk genes.

2. **Lifestyle factors**:

- Alcohol consumption: Women who drink more than two alcoholic beverages per day are at greater risk.
- Weight and obesity: Being overweight or obese, particularly after menopause, can increase the risk of breast cancer.

3. **Environmental factors**:

- **Radiation:** Exposure to ionising radiation, such as from X-rays or radiation therapy for other cancers, can increase the risk of breast cancer.
- **Oestrogen:** prolonged exposure to high levels of oestrogen can increase the risk of breast cancer.

Primary effects of breast cancer

- **Changes in size or shape of one or both breasts.** This can include swelling, lumps, or a feeling of fullness/heaviness.
- **Discharge from nipples**: Discharge from the nipples - clear, bloody, or occurring without squeezing.
- **Swelling in armpits**: Swelling or lumps in the armpit can be a sign of breast cancer, as lymph nodes in the armpit can be affected by the disease.
- **Dimpling on breast skin**: The skin on the breast may become dimpled or puckered, resembling the surface of an orange peel. This is often caused by the cancer invading the underlying tissues, so is usually a sign of advanced breast cancer.
- **Change in the appearance of the nipple**: The nipple may become inverted or flattened, or there may be a change in its texture or appearance.

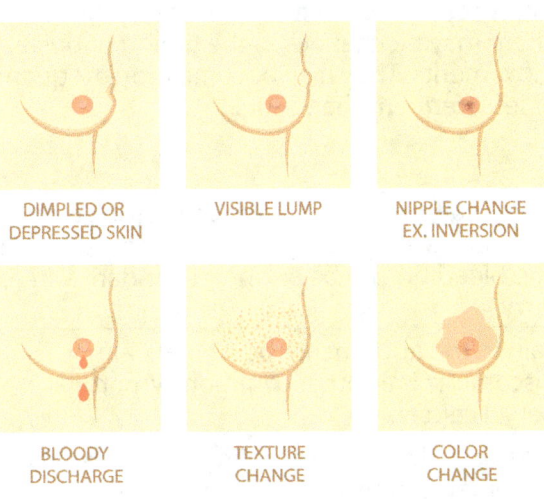

SYMPTOMS OF BREAST CANCER

DIMPLED OR DEPRESSED SKIN — VISIBLE LUMP — NIPPLE CHANGE EX. INVERSION

BLOODY DISCHARGE — TEXTURE CHANGE — COLOR CHANGE

Secondary effects of breast cancer

Metastasis occurs when cancer cells spread from the breast to other parts of the body. Once they reach a new location, these cells can invade surrounding tissues and grow into secondary tumours, known as **metastases**, in organs such as the bones, lungs, liver, and brain.

Metastasis (also known as Stage 4 cancer) can have a devastating impact on a person's health and can ultimately lead to organ failure and death:

- If breast cancer spreads to the lungs, it can interfere with breathing and lead to respiratory failure.
- If it spreads to the liver, it can damage the liver and impair its ability to filter toxins from the blood. This can lead to liver failure.
- If it spreads to the brain, it can cause neurological problems such as seizures, headaches, and cognitive decline.

Bowel cancer

Bowel cancer is a type of cancer that begins in the large intestine. A combination of genetic, lifestyle, and environmental factors are believed to play a role.

1. **Genetic factors**: Some individuals may have a genetic predisposition to bowel cancer. This means that they inherit genes that increase their risk of developing the disease.

2. **Lifestyle factors**:
   - Smoking: Smoking is a major risk factor for bowel cancer.
   - Consumption of red and processed meat: Eating large amounts of red and processed meat has been linked to an increased risk of bowel cancer.
   - Alcohol consumption: Excessive alcohol consumption can also increase the risk of bowel cancer.
   - Weight and obesity: Being overweight or obese can increase the risk of bowel cancer.

3. **Inflammatory bowel disease**: Individuals with inflammatory bowel disease, such as Crohn's disease or ulcerative colitis, have a higher risk of developing bowel cancer.

Primary effects of bowel cancer	Secondary effects of bowel cancer
Changes in faeces: This may include changes in the consistency of stools, such as becoming thicker, thinner, or more watery.	**Anaemia**: Internal bleeding or bleeding from the anus can lead to anaemia, a condition in which there is a decrease in the number of red blood cells. This can cause symptoms such as fatigue, weakness, and shortness of breath.
Changes in occurrence of defaecating: There may be changes in the timing of bowel movements. They may become more frequent or less frequent than usual.	**Musculoskeletal system**: The body may experience a loss of bone and muscle mass due to the cancer itself, the effects of treatment, or changes in diet and activity levels. This can lead to weakness, fatigue, and an increased risk of fractures.
Bleeding from the anus/blood in stool: Blood in the stool is a serious symptom of bowel cancer. The bleeding can be bright red, or dark and tarry.	**Metastasis**: This occurs when cancer cells spread from the bowel to other parts of the body. Metastasis can lead to organ failure and death. For example, if bowel cancer spreads to the liver, it can cause liver failure. If it spreads to the lungs, it can cause respiratory problems and difficulty breathing.
Pain in the abdomen: Abdominal pain or discomfort is another common symptom of bowel cancer.	
Bloating: Bloating or a feeling of fullness in the abdomen can be another symptom.	
Weight loss: Unexplained weight loss can be a sign of bowel cancer.	

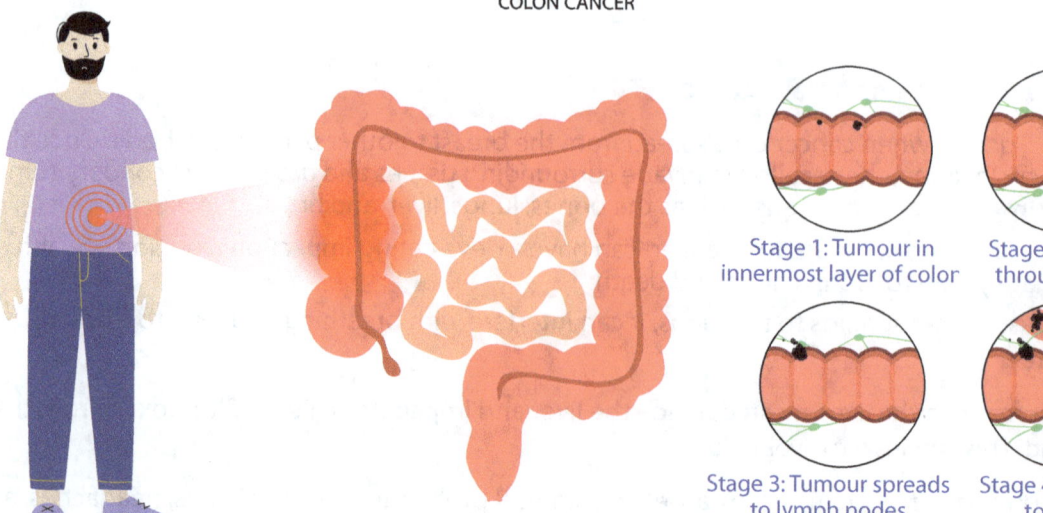

COLON CANCER

Stage 1: Tumour in innermost layer of color

Stage 2: Tumour grows through wall of colon

Stage 3: Tumour spreads to lymph nodes

Stage 4: Tumour spreads to other organs

Lung cancer

Lung cancer is a type of cancer that begins in the lungs. It is characterised by the uncontrolled growth of abnormal cells, which can form a tumour and potentially spread to other parts of the body. Like breast and bowel cancer, a combination of genetic, lifestyle, and environmental factors are believed to play a role:

1. **Genetic factors**: Some individuals may have a genetic predisposition to lung cancer, meaning they inherit genes that increase their risk of developing the disease.

2. **Lifestyle factors**: Smoking is the most significant risk factor for lung cancer and can significantly increase the risk of developing the disease. The longer you smoke and the more cigarettes you smoke, the higher your risk of lung cancer.

3. **Environmental factors**:
   - Passive smoking: Exposure to second-hand smoke can increase the risk of lung cancer, even if you do not smoke yourself.
   - Exposure to certain chemicals and substances: Exposure to chemicals and substances, such as arsenic and asbestos, can increase the risk of lung cancer. These substances are used in several occupations and industries, including mining, construction, and manufacturing.

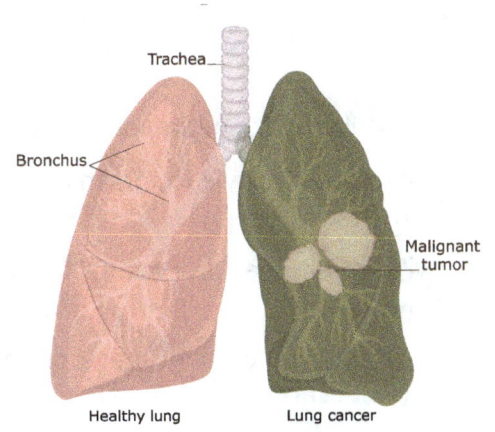

Primary effects of lung cancer	Secondary effects of lung cancer
Persistent cough: A persistent cough that does not go away is one of the most common symptoms of lung cancer. This cough may be dry or productive (produces phlegm).	**Anaemia**: Internal bleeding or coughing up blood can lead to anaemia, a condition in which there is a decrease in the number of red blood cells. This can cause symptoms such as fatigue, weakness, and shortness of breath.
Recurrent chest infections: This is because the cancer can weaken the lungs' ability to fight off infections.	**Blood clots**: Lung cancer can increase the risk of blood clots, which can lead to stroke (blood clots in the brain) or pulmonary embolism (blood clots in the lungs).
Coughing up blood: Coughing up blood is a serious symptom of lung cancer. This can occur when the cancer grows into the airways and causes bleeding.	**Loss of appetite and weight loss**: This can lead to malnutrition and weakness. This can be caused by the cancer itself, the effects of treatment, or changes in diet and activity levels.
Pain when breathing or coughing: Lung cancer can cause pain when breathing or coughing, especially if the tumour is pressing on nerves or other structures in the chest.	**Loss of bone and muscle mass**: This can be due to the cancer itself, the effects of treatment, or changes in diet and activity levels. This can lead to weakness, fatigue, and an increased risk of fractures.
	Metastasis: This occurs when cancer cells spread from the lungs to other parts of the body. For example, if lung cancer spreads to the brain, it can cause neurological problems such as seizures and cognitive decline.

> **Study Tips**
>
> The stages of cancer describe how far the cancer has progressed:
>
> - Stage 0: Abnormal cells are present but have not spread to nearby tissue. This is often considered pre-cancerous.
> - Stage 1: The cancer is small and contained within the organ where it started. It has not spread to lymph nodes or other parts of the body.
> - Stage 2: The cancer is larger than in Stage 1 and may have spread to nearby lymph nodes. It has not spread to distant parts of the body.
> - Stage 3: The cancer is larger and has likely spread to more surrounding tissue and/or a greater number of lymph nodes in the region. It has not spread to distant parts of the body.
> - Stage 4 (Metastatic): The cancer has spread from where it started to distant organs or tissues in the body. This is the most advanced stage.

Recap Questions

1. Describe two genetic factors that can increase a woman's risk of developing breast cancer.
2. Name two lifestyle factors that are associated with an increased risk of breast cancer and briefly explain why.
3. What are two environmental factors that may contribute to the development of breast cancer?
4. Describe four primary effects or noticeable changes in the breast that could be signs of breast cancer.
5. What is metastasis and how does it occur?
6. Explain the potential consequences of breast cancer metastasising (spreading) to the bones, lungs, liver, or brain.
7. How can the spread of breast cancer lead to organ failure?
8. Name one genetic factor that can increase an individual's risk of developing bowel cancer.
9. List three lifestyle factors that are associated with an increased risk of bowel cancer.
10. Name a pre-existing medical condition of the digestive system can increase the risk of bowel cancer.
11. Describe three primary effects or changes in bowel habits that could be signs of bowel cancer.
12. How can bowel cancer have a secondary effect on the cardiovascular system, and what condition can it lead to?
13. Explain how bowel cancer or its treatment can have a secondary effect on the musculoskeletal system.
14. Name the most significant lifestyle factor that dramatically increases the risk of developing lung cancer.
15. Describe two environmental factors, other than active smoking, that can increase the risk of lung cancer.
16. What is one of the most common primary effects of lung cancer?
17. Explain why individuals with lung cancer might experience recurrent chest infections.
18. Describe how can lung cancer have a secondary effect on the cardiovascular system, potentially leading to anaemia or blood clots.
19. Describe how lung cancer can have secondary effects on the digestive and musculoskeletal systems.
20. Name three organs commonly affected by the spread of lung cancer. What are the potential consequences of this spread?

> **Important terms!**
> Cancer risk-genes – Genes that raise the likelihood that a person will develop a certain type of cancer in their lifetime.
> Metastasis – When cancer spreads to different organs in different parts of the body from the original cancer.
> Tumour – A collection of abnormal cells. Tumours can be cancerous (also known as malignant) or non-cancerous (also known as benign).

Revision Quiz

1. Name three types of connective tissue and give the function of each type.
2. What is the role of glial cells in nervous tissue?
3. Where does aerobic respiration primarily take place within the cell?
4. What is the product of anaerobic respiration that causes muscle fatigue?
5. What is the primary mechanism the body uses to maintain homeostasis?
6. How does the body regulate temperature when it's too hot?
7. What hormones are involved in regulating blood sugar levels, and where are they produced?
8. What is osmoregulation, and which organ plays a key role in this process?
9. What is the function of the alveoli?
10. Describe the process of gas exchange in the lungs.
11. What muscles are involved in inhalation?
12. What hormones regulate water reabsorption in the kidneys?
13. Explain the role of antibodies in the immune response.
14. Describe the role of lymph nodes.
15. What are the roles of lymphatic capillaries?
16. What is the function of the small intestine?
17. Explain the role of the liver and gallbladder in digestion.
18. What are the functions of the ovaries?
19. What are the functions of the testes?
20. What are the roles of oestrogen and progesterone in the menstrual cycle?
21. Which blood vessels are primarily affected in coronary heart disease?
22. What is atherosclerosis, and how does it contribute to CHD?
23. What are the two main categories of stroke, and what are the differences between them?
24. Explain how a stroke affecting the left hemisphere of the brain might differ in its effects from a stroke affecting the right hemisphere.
25. What are the typical risk factors associated with type 2 diabetes?
26. How can dementia impact mood, behaviour, and personality?
27. In what ways can ABI impact motor skills and coordination?
28. How can a stroke impact the musculoskeletal system?

Assessment practice

1. State the causes of coronary heart disease. (2)
2. Explain how atherosclerosis leads to coronary heart disease. (5)
3. Describe and explain two secondary effects of coronary heart disease. (4)
4. Discuss the differences between a haemorrhagic stroke and an ischaemic stroke. (6)
5. Describe the impact a stroke has on the nervous system. (3)
6. Chronic obstructive pulmonary disorder (COPD) is a group of lung disorders that make it hard to breathe. Explain what is meant by the term 'chronic'. (2)
7. State the two main causes of COPD. (2)
8. Describe and explain how emphysema results in reduced gas exchange. (4)

> **Scenario**:
>
> Alex was diagnosed with COPD 10 years ago. Over the last year, she has lost a significant amount of weight. Her GP has also referred her to a cardiologist as she has been complaining of chest pains.

9. Discuss how COPD can affect Alex's digestive system and cardiovascular system. (9)
10. State three common triggers for asthma. (3)
11. Describe and explain two primary effects of asthma. (4)
12. Discuss the differences between Type 1 and Type 2 diabetes. (6)
13. Explain why Type 2 diabetes is classed as a lifestyle disease. (3)

> **Scenario**:
>
> Bailey has Type 1 diabetes. Bailey attends regular check ups at the hospital to ensure his condition is well managed.

14. Discuss the ways in which the effects of Type 1 diabetes can have an impact on Bailey's other body systems. (9)
15. Describe and explain three primary effects of dementia. (6)
16. Explain the difference between a traumatic and non-traumatic brain injury. (3)
17. Explain why a brain injury can lead to changes in personality. (4)
18. Explain how a combination of genetic, lifestyle, and environmental factors can lead to the development of breast cancer. (6)
19. Explain what is meant by metastatic cancer. (2)
20. Describe three primary effects of bowel cancer. (3)
21. Describe the impact bowel cancer can have on the musculoskeletal system. (3)

> **Scenario**:
>
> Frankie was diagnosed with lung cancer last year. They are attending an appointment with dietitian due to weight loss and have an appointment the following week with the cardiovascular unit.

22. Discuss how Frankie's lung cancer may affect the functioning of the digestive system and other body systems. (9)

www.ingramcontent.com/pod-product-compliance
Lightning Source LLC
Chambersburg PA
CBHW081103070526
44584CB00021B/3186